GLUTEN FREE BAKING

Gluten Free, Healthy, Easy and Delicious Recipes

(Simple and Delicious Gluten-free Recipes for a Healthy Lifestyle)

Michael Hastings

Published by Sharon Lohan

Gluten Free Baking: Gluten Free, Healthy, Easy and Delicious Recipes (Simple and Delicious Gluten-free Recipes for a Healthy Lifestyle)

ISBN 978-1-990334-16-0

Legal & Disclaimer

The information contained in this book is not designed to replace or take the place of any form of medicine or professional medical advice. The information in this book has been provided for educational and entertainment purposes only.

Table of contents

Part 1

Introduction

I want to thank you and congratulate you for downloading my book.

Gluten-Free foods has become a necessity now a days, you have to bar gluten out from your diet plan to stay healthy. With the increase of people suffering from celiac disease and food allergies, it's wise to adapt gluten free food for a healthy family.

Life is very busy now a day, everybody wants to eat fresh and healthy food which is easy to prepare. This book will help you to achieve more balance in your health.

So, I personally took the initiative to write a cookbook for you containing Gluten-Free recipes. This book contains mouth-watering, easy to *make gluten-free recipes for breakfast, lunch, dinner, soup and desserts,* for you to cook and enjoy. Only Gluten-Free ingredients are used in my recipes.

All about Gluten

What is Gluten?

Gluten is the mixture of two different proteins, gliadin and glutenin, found in cereal grain which affects in the elastic texture of dough. Gluten is found in Rye, Wheat, Barley and any foods made with these cereal grains.

Why is gluten bad?

Some people are intolerant to gluten, which means they are prone to an abnormal immune response when their bodies' breakdown cereal grains with gluten during digestion. This gluten intolerance is well-known as Celiac Disease.

When someone suffering from celiac disease consume food containing gluten, the immune response which damages their intestine is triggered which prevents them from absorbing vital nutrients from the food.

For people having gluten intolerance, doctors typically recommend a gluten-free diet plan. People must avoid eating any food and ingredients that contains gluten.

"Eat Healthy and Gluten-Free food"

Complete List of Gluten Free Food

Fruits

Acai	Apples	Apricot	Bananas
Blackberries	Blueberries	Cantaloupe	Carob
Cherry	Cranberries	Currants	Dates
Figs	Grapes	Guava	Honeydew Melon
Kiwi	Kumquat	Lemons	Limes
Passion Fruit	Peaches	Pears	Pineapples
Plantains	Plums	Persimmons	Quince
Raspberries	Strawberries	Tamarind	Tangerines
Watermelons	Mangoes	Oranges	Papaya

Vegetables

Acorn	Agar	Alfalfa	Algae
Arrowroot	Artichoke	Arugula	Asparagus
Avocado	Beans	Broccoli	Watercress
Cauliflower	Cabbage	Carrots	Celery
Corn	Cucumber	Eggplant	Garlic
Green Beans	Kale	Lettuce	Mushrooms
Okra	Onions	Parsley	Peas
Peppers	Potatoes (white and sweet)	Pumpkins	Radish
Spinach	Squash	Turnips	

Meats

Venison	Beef	Buffalo	Chicken
Duck	Goat	Goose	Lamb
Pork	Rabbit	Snake	Turkey
Quail	Veal		

Eggs and Dairy Products

Butter (be sure it has no additives)	Casein	Cheese	Cream
Eggs	Milk	Sour Cream	Yogurt- plain and not flavored
Whey			

Flour, Grains, and Wheat

Almond Flour	Amaranth	Arrowroot	Bean flour
Besan	Brown rice	Brown rice flour	Buckwheat
Cassava	Corn flour	Corn meal	Corn starch
Cottonseed	Dal	Flaxseed	Millet
Pea Flour	Polenta	Popcorn – without coating	Potato flour
Quinoa	Rice	Sago	Soy Flour
Tapioca Flour	Taro Flour	Tef	Yucca

Other gluten free foods

Baking Soda	Herbs	Honey	Jam
Jelly	Juice	Nuts	Oils
Seeds	Spices (most)	Syrup	Vanilla
Vinegar	Vitamins	Wine	Xanthan Gum

1 Gluten-Free Breakfast Recipes

Minted Cabbage Salad

Serves - 2
Cooks In - 35 minutes
Difficulty - Super easy

Ingredients

- 2 spring onions
- 1 large carrot
- 250 grams of red and white cabbage each
- ½ handful of mixed seeds
- 2 cloves of garlic
- 15 leaves of fresh mint
- 100 ml milk
- 2 spring onions
- 2 tablespoons extra virgin olive oil
- 1 tablespoons white vinegar

Method

1. Shred both the cabbages and spring onion finely, peel off the carrot and slice it into small pieces.
2. Place all of them in a bowl and mix them.
3. Take a pan put it on the gas stove. Pour milk and then add cloves of peeled garlic and allow it to simmer.
4. Cook it for 10 min. until the cloves soften.

5. Pour the milk into the blender jar, add vinegar, olive oil (you can use 1 teaspoon of mustard oil for taste) and blend it.
6. Scatter the mixture over the veggies.
7. Add a pinch of black pepper and salt as per taste.
8. Heat the seeds in a dry pan for 1 min.
9. Scatter them over the veggies.
10. Garnish them with finely chopped mint

Nutrition Facts	
Serving Size 426 g	
Amount Per Serving	
Calories 242	Calories from Fat 139
	% Daily Value*
Total Fat 15.4g	24%
Saturated Fat 2.7g	14%
Trans Fat 0.0g	
Cholesterol 4mg	1%
Sodium 102mg	4%
Potassium 704mg	20%
Total Carbohydrates 24.5g	8%
Dietary Fiber 8.5g	34%
Sugars 12.8g	
Protein 6.2g	
Vitamin A 137% •	Vitamin C 169%
Calcium 22% •	Iron 15%
Nutrition Grade A	
* Based on a 2000 calorie diet	

leaves .Then ENJOY!

Zucchini spring salad with Dill

Serves - 2
Cooks In- 10 minutes
Difficulty - Super easy

Ingredients

- extra virgin olive oil
- 5-6 piece of asparagus
- 5-6 pieces of radishes
- 4 baby zucchini
- 15 leaves of fresh mint
- ½ a bunch of fresh dill
- 1 lemon

Method

1. Take a bowl and pour water in it.
2. Peel the Radish, Zucchini and asparagus and trim veggies into ribbon shaped pieces.
3. Place the veggies into the water.
4. Take mint leaves and dill, chop it finely and place in a bowl.
5. Season it well with olive oil, pinch of pepper, salt and lemon juice.
6. Take out the veggies from the water and dry it.

7. Place the veggies in the bowl with the seasoned mint leaves and dill.
8. Serve it after tossing it properly.

Nutrition Facts

Serving Size 150 g

Amount Per Serving

Calories 99	Calories from Fat 67
	% Daily Value*
Total Fat 7.4g	11%
Saturated Fat 1.1g	5%
Cholesterol 0mg	0%
Sodium 36mg	1%
Potassium 490mg	14%
Total Carbohydrates 8.4g	3%
Dietary Fiber 3.5g	14%
Sugars 2.4g	
Protein 3.1g	
Vitamin A 21% •	Vitamin C 34%
Calcium 13% •	Iron 26%

Nutrition Grade A

* Based on a 2000 calorie diet

Fruity Gluten-Free Pancakes

Serves - 2
Cooks In- 15 minutes
Difficulty- Super easy

Ingredients

- 1 Apple
- 1 Banana
- 1 Pear
- ¼ Pomegranate (peel off the seeds)
- Handful of oats
- 4 tablespoon honey
- 2 Eggs
- 100 grams Cheese
- Groundnut oil
- 4 tablespoon yoghurt(Fat Free)
- Pinch of Baking powder
- 1 teaspoon sugar
- ½ teaspoon salt
- Almond butter
- 2/3 cup of Almond milk
- 4 Common fig

Method

1. Take all the dry pancake ingredients in a bowl.
2. Take a separate bowl, place almond milk cheese, oats and eggs and whisk it properly
3. Make sure it is smooth .Then pour the dry ingredients into the bowl with the whisked egg cheese and milk and then use blender to whisk it properly.
4. Slice the common figs, cut or grate the pear and apple in to small pieces and take pomegranate seeds in a bowl.
5. Take a frying pan heat it over a medium temperature, pour 1 teaspoon oil .
6. Take the prepared mixture and drop it into the pan.
7. Cook it for 3-4 minutes, flip it properly, and again cook it till the colour is light golden.
8. Transfer it to the plate, Dress it with the sliced fruits, butter, and yogurt and pour some honey.

Nutrition Facts

Serving Size 530 g

Amount Per Serving

Calories 964	Calories from Fat 486
	% Daily Value*
Total Fat 54.0g	83%
Saturated Fat 30.9g	155%
Trans Fat 0.0g	
Cholesterol 218mg	73%
Sodium 993mg	41%
Potassium 1034mg	30%
Total Carbohydrates 102.6g	34%
Dietary Fiber 10.7g	43%
Sugars 68.3g	
Protein 27.9g	

Vitamin A 16%	•	Vitamin C 32%	
Calcium 51%	•	Iron 27%	

Nutrition Grade B

* Based on a 2000 calorie diet

Breakfast Quinoa with Walnuts and Blueberries

Serves - 2
Cooks In- 15 minutes
Difficulty- Super easy

Ingredients

- ¼ cup Blueberries (fresh)
- 1 tablespoon Walnuts (chopped)
- ½ cup Quinoa (uncooked)
- 1 tablespoon Almond butter
- 1 cup Milk
- 1 tablespoon Cinnamon

Method

1. Take a fine mesh strainer; place the quinoa, rinse and drain.
2. In a saucepan mix quinoa and milk, boil it.
3. Reduce the heat and cook it for 15-20 minutes until the quinoa is tender and the milk is absorbed.
4. Remove it from the burner.

5. Add Cinnamon, Almond butter and Walnuts into the saucepan and mix it thoroughly.
6. Keep it for some time to cool.
7. Take it out & serve it with fresh Blueberries.

Nutrition Facts

Serving Size 198 g

Amount Per Serving	
Calories 311	Calories from Fat 108

	% Daily Value*
Total Fat 12.0g	18%
Saturated Fat 2.4g	12%
Trans Fat 0.0g	
Cholesterol 10mg	3%
Sodium 60mg	3%
Potassium 419mg	12%
Total Carbohydrates 40.4g	13%
Dietary Fiber 5.8g	23%
Sugars 7.4g	
Protein 12.9g	

Vitamin A 1%	•	Vitamin C 5%	
Calcium 22%	•	Iron 16%	

Nutrition Grade B+
* Based on a 2000 calorie diet

Blueberries Oatmeal Breakfast

Serves - 4
Cooks In- 30 minutes
Difficulty- Super easy

Ingredients

- Salt ¼ Teaspoon
- Walnuts ¼ cup ,Chopped
- Blueberries 1 cup
- Walnuts ¼ cup, Chopped
- Brown sugar
- Water 3 cups
- Oatmeal 1 cup, Uncooked
- Cinnamon ½ teaspoon
- Ground Nutmeg ¼ teaspoon

Method

1. Take a saucepan & heat water, oatmeal, nutmeg, cinnamon, and add salt to boiling. Reduce the heat and simmer for 25 to 30 minutes, stir occasionally until the oatmeal softens by absorbing water. Remove the saucepan.

2. Take the blueberries and boil for 2-3 minutes until they are hot. Mix them with oatmeal.
3. Now Serve it in a bowl and dress it with chopped walnut and sprinkle brown sugar.

Nutrition Facts

Serving Size 506 g

Amount Per Serving	
Calories 410	Calories from Fat 193

	% Daily Value*
Total Fat 21.5g	33%
Saturated Fat 1.6g	8%
Trans Fat 0.0g	
Cholesterol 0mg	0%
Sodium 306mg	13%
Potassium 360mg	11%
Total Carbohydrates 46.3g	15%
Dietary Fiber 8.4g	33%
Sugars 12.4g	
Protein 13.5g	

Vitamin A 0%	•	Vitamin C 20%
Calcium 8%	•	Iron 21%

Nutrition Grade B+

* Based on a 2000 calorie diet

Mango and Blueberry Pancakes

Serves – 25 (Small pancakes)
Cooks In- 30 minutes
Difficulty- Super easy

Ingredients

- Salt
- Cooking oil
- Nut or Almond butter
- Oats -230 grams
- Blueberries – 150 grams, optional
- Water 2 cups
- Banana -230 grams (2 Pieces)
- Mango – 150 grams (5-6 slice)

Method

1. Take the peeled banana, mango slices, oats , almond butter, water and salt in a blender and whisk it for 1 minute until the mix is even and smooth.
2. Place the mixture in a bowl, add blueberries and leave it for 3-4 minutes so it absorbs some fluids.
3. Heat a non-sticky pan and pour some oil in it.Once the pan is hot start pouring small amount of mixture

to the pan . (Amount of mixture depends upon the size of pancake you want)

4. Cook it for 2-3 minutes until the crust is light golden. Flip the pancake and do the same.
5. Once both sides are properly cooked it's ready to be served.
6. Serve it hot.

Nutrition Facts

Serving Size 636 g

Amount Per Serving

Calories 704	Calories from Fat 136
	% Daily Value*
Total Fat 15.1g	23%
Saturated Fat 2.2g	11%
Cholesterol 0mg	0%
Sodium 3505mg	146%
Potassium 1066mg	30%
Total Carbohydrates 129.1g	43%
Dietary Fiber 18.1g	72%
Sugars 33.9g	
Protein 19.0g	

Vitamin A 13%	•	Vitamin C 71%
Calcium 10%	•	Iron 37%

Nutrition Grade A
* Based on a 2000 calorie diet

Lemony Muffins with Poppy seeds

Nutrition Facts

Serving Size 164 g	

Amount Per Serving	
Calories 525	Calories from Fat 322

	% Daily Value*
Total Fat 35.8g	55%
Saturated Fat 7.9g	39%
Trans Fat 0.0g	
Cholesterol 246mg	82%
Sodium 1447mg	60%
Potassium 151mg	4%
Total Carbohydrates 45.1g	15%
Dietary Fiber 5.7g	23%
Sugars 37.1g	
Protein 11.3g	

Vitamin A 6%	•	Vitamin C 6%	
Calcium 10%	•	Iron 20%	

Nutrition Grade C
* Based on a 2000 calorie diet

Serves – 20 (mini muffins)
Cooks In- 30 minutes
Difficulty- Super easy

Ingredients

- Lemon Zest 1 Tablespoon
- Poppy seeds 1 Tablespoon
- Honey ¼ cup
- Eggs (3 Large Size)
- Coconut Flour ¼ cup
- Baking Soda ¼ Teaspoon
- Salt
- Olive oil ¼ cup

Method

1. Take a blender , mix coconut flour ,baking soda and salt together properly

2. Add eggs, lemon zest, poppy seeds, honey, and olive oil and whisk it.
3. Your batter is ready, take one tablespoon batter at a time and place into muffin cups.
4. Set the oven for 350 degrees and bake for 8-12 minutes.
5. Cool it and Serve with icing on top.

Crunchy Almond Granola

Serves – 15
Cooks In- 30 minutes
Difficulty- Super easy

Ingredients:

- Salt - ½ Tablespoon
- Cooking Oil - ¼ cup
- Vanilla - 1 Tablespoon
- Rolled oats - 4 cups
- Vanilla bean - 1 tablespoon
- Almond - 1 ½ cups , Sliced
- Brown sugar - ½ cup
- Honey - ¼ cup
- Ground Cinnamon - ½ tablespoon

Method

1. Take Salt, Rolled Oats, Vanilla bean, Brown sugar, Ground Cinnamon in a bowl and mix them together.
2. Take a saucepan pour oil, honey, and vanilla and warm it over low heat for ½ minutes.
3. Then pour the mixture over the rolled oat and bean mixture. Properly mix it.
4. Spread the mixture over baking sheet lined with parchment.

5. Set oven temperature at 300 degrees for 40 minutes.
6. Keep stirring every 10 minutes or so.
7. When the granola is golden in colour, it is done.
8. Remove it from the oven and allow it to cool.
9. Enjoy the crispy healthy granola.
10. Store leftovers in an airtight container.

Nutrition Facts

Serving Size 361 g

Amount Per Serving	
Calories 1,586	Calories from Fat 662
	% Daily Value*
Total Fat 73.6g	113%
Saturated Fat 8.6g	43%
Trans Fat 0.0g	
Cholesterol 0mg	0%
Sodium 1780mg	74%
Potassium 1210mg	35%
Total Carbohydrates 204.6g	68%
Dietary Fiber 26.4g	106%
Sugars 76.1g	
Protein 36.8g	
Vitamin A 0% •	Vitamin C 24%
Calcium 33% •	Iron 57%

Nutrition Grade B-
* Based on a 2000 calorie diet

Quinoa Breakfast Porridge with Honey

```
                Nutrition Facts
         Serving Size 546 g
         Amount Per Serving
         Calories 1,012            Calories from Fat 311
                                        % Daily Value*
         Total Fat 34.6g                          53%
            Saturated Fat 26.0g                   130%
            Trans Fat 0.0g
         Cholesterol 0mg                           0%
         Sodium 39mg                               2%
         Potassium 1637mg                         47%
         Total Carbohydrates 173.1g               58%
            Dietary Fiber 15.3g                    61%
            Sugars 90.4g
         Protein 18.7g
         Vitamin A 0%        •        Vitamin C 36%
         Calcium 13%         •           Iron 52%
         Nutrition Grade C+
         * Based on a 2000 calorie diet
```

Serves – 2
Cooks In- 30 minutes
Difficulty- Super easy

Ingredients

- Water – 1 cup
- Almond Milk – 1 cups
- Quinoa - 1 cup
- Honey – 2 Tablespoon
- Ground Cinnamon - 1 teaspoon
- Blueberries – 200 grams
- Raisins – 200 grams

Method

1. Take a small saucepan, boil 1 cup water and add 1 cup quinoa.

2. Add 1 teaspoon cinnamon cover the saucepan and boil for 15 minutes.
3. Remove the cover, add 1 cup almond milk and stir it.
4. Reduce the heat and simmer for 10 minutes.
5. The porridge must be thickened by now.
6. Stir in some honey.
7. Dress it with blueberries and raisins...and enjoy!

Omelet Pepperoncino

Nutrition Facts

Nutrition Facts	
Serving Size 177 g	
Amount Per Serving	
Calories 167	Calories from Fat 98
	% Daily Value*
Total Fat 10.8g	17%
Saturated Fat 3.2g	16%
Cholesterol 11mg	4%
Sodium 1865mg	78%
Potassium 296mg	8%
Total Carbohydrates 8.8g	3%
Dietary Fiber 2.5g	10%
Sugars 4.6g	
Protein 9.3g	
Vitamin A 38%	Vitamin C 113%
Calcium 11%	Iron 6%
Nutrition Grade B	
* Based on a 2000 calorie diet	

Serves – 2
Cooks In- 30 minutes
Difficulty- Super easy

Ingredients

- Onion – 100 Grams , Chopped
- Fresh Mint – 10 leaves
- Salt - ½ Tablespoon
- Black Pepper – ¼ Teaspoon
- Bell Pepper – 100 grams. Sliced
- Olive oil – 1 Tablespoon
- Egg White – 3 pieces
- Cheese - 3 Tablespoon

Method

26

1. Take a Fry pan pour olive oil and fry onions until they are translucent.
2. Add sliced Bell Peppers.
3. After Bell Pepper softens, pour in egg white.
4. Wait until it sets.
5. Add Cheese and sprinkle salt, black pepper and mint leaves.
6. Fold Omelet and serve it on a plate

2 Gluten- Free Lunch Recipes

Cheesy Chicken salad

Serves – 2
Cooks In- 20 minutes
Preparation time - 35 min
Difficulty- Easy

Ingredients

- Olive oil – 4 tablespoon
- Cheese – 1 ½ oz.
- Salt – ½ tablespoon
- Boneless Chicken Breast – 10 oz.
- Eggs – 3 pieces
- Bacon Rashers – 10 grams
- Baby Lettuce -1 piece ,Chopped
- Gluten free French Bread – 8 slices

Method

1. Take non-sticky frying pan pour oil and cook the chicken for 5-6 minutes over medium heat. Flip side until chicken is cooked properly. Remove it from the pan. Slice it into strips.
2. In a saucepan place eggs and boil it for 5-7 minutes. Cover it, sprinkle pinch of salt to increase the boiling process faster .Peel the egg shell and slice it into small pieces.
3. Cook the bacon in the frying pan for 2-3 minutes, until it's golden.
4. Grill the French bread, cut it into small pieces.
5. On a plate place the bread, lettuce, chicken slices, eggs and bacon, toss it.
6. Sprinkle cheese to dress.

Nutrition Facts

Serving Size 472 g

Amount Per Serving

Calories 1,197	Calories from Fat 632
	% Daily Value*
Total Fat 70.2g	108%
Saturated Fat 24.2g	121%
Trans Fat 0.0g	
Cholesterol 400mg	133%
Sodium 3446mg	144%
Potassium 495mg	14%
Total Carbohydrates 81.0g	27%
Dietary Fiber 4.1g	16%
Sugars 0.7g	
Protein 64.4g	

Vitamin A 18%	•	Vitamin C 62%
Calcium 37%	•	Iron 18%

Nutrition Grade D+
* Based on a 2000 calorie diet

Crispy Chicken Nuggets

```
Nutrition Facts
Serving Size 535 g
Amount Per Serving
Calories 1,298          Calories from Fat 390
                              % Daily Value*
Total Fat 43.3g                          67%
  Saturated Fat 4.9g                     24%
  Trans Fat 0.0g
Cholesterol 377mg                       126%
Sodium 1733mg                            72%
Potassium 960mg                          27%
Total Carbohydrates 103.6g               35%
  Dietary Fiber 1.1g                      4%
  Sugars 1.4g
Protein 119.5g
Vitamin A 4%           •      Vitamin C 1%
Calcium 9%             •          Iron 32%
Nutrition Grade B-
* Based on a 2000 calorie diet
```

Serves – 2

Cooks In- 20 minutes

Preparation time - 40 min

Difficulty- Easy

Ingredients

- Garlic Salt – 1 Teaspoon
- Salt – 1 Teaspoon
- Egg – 1 piece
- Chicken Breast – 4 Pieces
- Olive oil – 4 Tablespoon
- Bread Crumbs -4 Tablespoon
- Black Pepper
- Chili Powder -1/4 Teaspoon
- Gluten free Flour – 240 grams

Method

1. Take a bowl combine Flour, Salt, Garlic Salt, pepper, bread crumbs and toss it properly.

2. In another bowl break the egg and prepare liquid egg by segregating the yoke. You can use the yoke if you want. Stir it properly.

3. Take the chicken breast and slice it into thin strips.

4. Dip the chicken first into the liquid egg.

5. Then cover the chicken with flour mixture prepared earlier. You can repeat the dipping procedure for thicker crust .

6. On an oiled baking sheet lined with parchment pour, place the dipped chicken.

7. Bake at 450 degree Fahrenheit for 15 -20 minutes.

8. Flip the Chicken nuggets after 8-10 minutes and oil them again.

9. Your Chicken Nuggets with crispy crust are ready to be served...Enjoy

Lemon-Paprika Fried Salmon

Nutrition Facts

Serving Size 651 g	
Amount Per Serving	
Calories 588	Calories from Fat 267
	% Daily Value*
Total Fat 29.6g	46%
Saturated Fat 4.3g	22%
Trans Fat 0.0g	
Cholesterol 154mg	51%
Sodium 252mg	10%
Potassium 2059mg	59%
Total Carbohydrates 12.9g	4%
Dietary Fiber 4.0g	16%
Sugars 7.3g	
Protein 71.0g	
Vitamin A 66% •	Vitamin C 73%
Calcium 17% •	Iron 26%
Nutrition Grade B+	
* Based on a 2000 calorie diet	

Serves – 4

Cooks In- 20 minutes

Preparation time - 5 min

Difficulty- Easy

Ingredients

- Lime Juice – 2 tablespoon
- Salt
- Clove Garlic – 1 Piece , Minced
- Medium tomatoes – 4 Piece , Halved
- Black pepper
- Salmon Steaks – 700 grams (2-4 Pieces)
- Cooking oil – 1 Tablespoon
- Smoked Paprika – ½ Tablespoon
- Lettuce – 1 piece , Chopped
- Cumin – ½ Tablespoon

Method

1. Wash and dry salmon steaks.
2. Mix salt, pepper, paprika and cumin.
3. Rub the mixture on both sides of steaks properly.
4. Take a frying pan , pour oil and heat it over medium heat
5. Add the salmon steaks and halved tomatoes and garlic to frying pan; cook it for 6-7 minutes. Flip sides of salmon until it's golden and tomatoes and garlic are tender.
6. Take a plate place lettuce, tomatoes and salmon steaks.
7. Serve it hot...

Beef Chili with Beans

Serves – 4
Cooks In- 20 minutes
Preparation time - 10 min
Difficulty- Easy

Ingredients

- Salt - 1 Tablespoon
- Water – 2 cups
- Clove Garlic – 2-3 Piece , Minced
- Kidney beans – 40 grams , Rinsed and Drained
- Medium tomatoes – 4 Piece , Halved
- Black pepper – 1 Tablespoon
- Garlic Powder – 1 Tablespoon
- Minced Beef – 900 grams (2-4 Pieces)
- Smoked Paprika – 1 Tablespoon
- Lettuce – 1 piece , Chopped
- Cumin – 2 Tablespoon
- Butter – 1 tablespoon
- Onion -1 Large, Diced
- Chili powder – 3 Tablespoon
- Canned tomatoes – 1 (28oz) can ,Crushed

Method

1. Take a large frying pan with lid, heat it over medium temperature.
2. Melt butter and add diced onion, garlic and tomatoes . Fry it until it softens for about 2- 3 minutes.
3. Add Beef to the frying pan and stir it until it is brown.
4. Mix pepper, garlic powder, cumin, chili powder with 3 tablespoons water, and pour the mixture over the frying pan as it is still cooking. Toss it well.
5. Add water and beans, bring it to boil.
6. Reduce the heat.
7. Simmer the meat for about 20-25 minutes or until the liquid vaporizes, stir it every 5 minutes.
1. Add salt and pepper to taste.

Turkey Delight with Smoked Paprika

```
                Nutrition Facts
        Serving Size 343 g

        Amount Per Serving
        Calories 341             Calories from Fat 149
                                        % Daily Value*
        Total Fat 16.5g                          25%
            Saturated Fat 3.4g                    17%
            Trans Fat 0.0g
        Cholesterol 76mg                         25%
        Sodium 1179mg                            49%
        Potassium 842mg                          24%
        Total Carbohydrates 15.5g                 5%
            Dietary Fiber 3.7g                    15%
            Sugars 8.6g
        Protein 31.3g

        Vitamin A 37%        •      Vitamin C 42%
        Calcium 5%           •            Iron 70%
        Nutrition Grade A-
        * Based on a 2000 calorie diet
```

Serves – 5
Cooks In- 20 minutes
Preparation time - 15 min
Difficulty- Easy

Ingredients

- Cooking Oil – 4 tablespoon
- Salt - ½ Tablespoon
- Water – 1 cups
- Clove Garlic – 2-3 Piece , Minced
- Black pepper – 1 Tablespoon
- Minced Turkey – 500 grams
- Smoked Paprika – ¼ Tablespoon
- Cumin – ½ Tablespoon
- Onion – ½ Large, Chopped
- Chili powder – ½ Tablespoon
- Canned tomatoes – 1 ½ cup ,Crushed

36

- Tomatoes Sauce -1 ½ cup
- Sweet Potato – 1 Medium size peeled and chopped small.
- Coriander Leaves – ½ Bunch, Sliced
- Yogurt – 1 ½ Tablespoon.

Method

1. Take a large skillet; pour 2 tablespoon cooking oil and cook turkey over medium heat until its brown. Season it with salt, pepper and cumin.
2. Add onion and garlic and cook it for 3-4 minutes over medium heat.
3. Add sweet potato, chili powder, tomatoes , water , paprika and tomato sauce.
4. Cover skillet and simmer for 20-25 minutes over medium heat. Stir every 5 minutes.
5. Potato will be softened by this time.
6. Dress it with yogurt and coriander leaves.
7. Serve It.

Rosemary Roasted Lamb

Nutrition Facts

Serving Size 198 g	

Amount Per Serving	
Calories 426	Calories from Fat 197

	% Daily Value*
Total Fat 21.9g	34%
Saturated Fat 6.0g	30%
Cholesterol 162mg	54%
Sodium 1553mg	65%
Potassium 637mg	18%
Total Carbohydrates 3.8g	1%
Dietary Fiber 0.7g	3%
Sugars 0.6g	
Protein 51.2g	

Vitamin A 0%	•	Vitamin C 1%
Calcium 4%	•	Iron 26%

Nutrition Grade B-
* Based on a 2000 calorie diet

Serves – 5

Cooks In- 20 minutes

Preparation time - 10 min

Difficulty- Easy

Ingredients

- Garlic Powder – 1 Tablespoon
- Bread Crumbs – 2 Tablespoon
- Boneless Lamb Loin – 900 grams ,Sliced
- Rosemary – 1 Tablespoon
- Salt – 1 tablespoon
- Black Pepper – ¼ tablespoon
- Olive oil – 3 Tablespoon

Method

1. Marinate lamb with 1 tablespoon oil, salt & pepper. Toss it properly.
2. Take a skillet & add 1 tablespoon of oil and heat at medium-heat.

3. Place the lamb onto the skillet for 30 seconds each side, transfer it to a
4. pan.
5. Prepare a mixture of rosemary, garlic powder, olive oil and bread crumbs in a bowl. Rub the mixture onto the lamb generously.
6. Take the lamb to the oven and roast it for 15 -20 minutes at 160 degrees.
7. Transfer the lamb to a cutting board , and cut into ½ inch thick slices.
8. Serve it with some bread.

Baked Garlic Meatballs

Serves – 4
Cooks In- 20 minutes
Preparation time - 15 min
Difficulty- Easy

Ingredients

- Cinnamon- ¼ teaspoon
- Salt – 1 Teaspoon
- Ground Beef – 250 grams
- Ground Pork – 250 grams
- Olive oil
- Onion – 1 small piece
- Carrot - 1 Small piece , peeled and sliced
- Garlic – 2 cloves ,Peeled and sliced
- Vinegar – 1 tablespoon
- Tomato Ketchup – ½ cup
- Parsley – ¼ cup ,Chopped finely
- Organic Molasses – 1 Tablespoon
- Bread Crumbs – ½ cup

Method

1. Take a large mixing bowl, stir beef and pork.

2. Mix carrot, garlic and onion pieces into a food processor, pulsing for some time it gets a finely diced texture. Keep it aside.
3. Take another mixing bowl; stir together the pork and beef.
4. Add carrot and onion mixture along with ketchup, pepper, molasses, parsley, vinegar, bread crumbs and salt into the bowl of meat. Mix them gently.
5. Now start making small meat balls from the mixture you made. Take some oil on your hands.
6. In a baking sheet with parchment pour, grease it with some oil and then place the meatballs.
7. Bake them for about 20 minutes into pre-heated oven at 350ºF.
8. Serve it hot and ENJOY...

Nutrition Facts

Serving Size 218 g

Amount Per Serving	
Calories 349	Calories from Fat 94

	% Daily Value*
Total Fat 10.5g	16%
Saturated Fat 2.9g	14%
Trans Fat 0.0g	
Cholesterol 101mg	34%
Sodium 1105mg	46%
Potassium 825mg	24%
Total Carbohydrates 24.8g	8%
Dietary Fiber 1.6g	6%
Sugars 11.9g	
Protein 38.1g	

Vitamin A 54%	•	Vitamin C 20%
Calcium 6%	•	Iron 77%

Nutrition Grade A
* Based on a 2000 calorie diet

Hot Pepper Chicken

Serves – 2
Cooks In- 20 minutes
Preparation time - 10 min
Difficulty- Easy

Ingredients

- Salt – ¼ Tablespoon
- Pepper – ¼ Tablespoon
- Chicken Breast – 2 piece , Halves
- Olive oil – ½ cup
- Onion powder – ¼ Tablespoon
- Bread or Cornflake Crumbs – ½ cup
- Cornmeal – ¼ cup

Method

1. Preheat oven at 350ºF.
2. Cut the chicken breast halves into nugget size pieces.
3. Take a bowl and mix salt, pepper, onion powder, crumbs, and cornmeal   all together.

4. Now, take the chicken and coat the pieces with olive oil.
5. Coat the chicken with the mixture, toss it properly.
6. In a baking sheet with parchment pour, grease it with some oil and then place the chicken nuggets.
7. Bake it for 15- 20 minutes in preheated oven.
8. Serve it with a sauce.

Nutrition Facts

Serving Size 254 g

Amount Per Serving

Calories 798	Calories from Fat 517
	% Daily Value*
Total Fat 57.4g	88%
Saturated Fat 7.3g	37%
Trans Fat 0.0g	
Cholesterol 147mg	49%
Sodium 1136mg	47%
Potassium 507mg	14%
Total Carbohydrates 17.4g	6%
Dietary Fiber 1.6g	6%
Sugars 0.8g	
Protein 57.4g	

Vitamin A 1%	•	Vitamin C 1%
Calcium 5%	•	Iron 19%

Nutrition Grade C+

* Based on a 2000 calorie diet

Lemony Fish Fillets with Rice

Serves – 4
Cooks In- 20 minutes
Preparation time - 10 min
Difficulty- Easy

Ingredients

- Olive oil – ¼ cup
- Lemon – ½ piece
- Fish Fillet – 2- 4
- Pepper – ¼ tablespoon
- Salt – ¼ tablespoon
- Parsley – ½ bunch , Chopped
- Paprika Powder – ¼ teaspoon
- Broth – 1 ½ Cup
- Long Grain Rice – ½ cup

Method

1. Preheat oven for 375 degree F.
2. Grease the Fish Fillet with oil.
3. Season the fish fillet with salt and pepper, sprinkle paprika powder.

4. Take a baking sheet with parchment pour, grease it with oil.
5. Take a saucepan and pour broth, heat it over medium heat to boil.
6. Stir rice in the saucepan; simmer it for 20 minutes until the rice is tender.
7. Place the baking sheet into the oven for 10 minutes, until it is light brown.
8. Serve the rice onto a plate, top it with fish fillets
9. Squeeze some lemon juice and sprinkle parsley on to the fish fillets

Nutrition Facts

Serving Size 189 g

Amount Per Serving	
Calories 320	Calories from Fat 171
	% Daily Value*
Total Fat 19.0g	29%
Saturated Fat 3.3g	16%
Cholesterol 15mg	5%
Sodium 975mg	41%
Potassium 338mg	10%
Total Carbohydrates 28.1g	9%
Dietary Fiber 1.3g	5%
Sugars 0.5g	
Protein 10.6g	

Vitamin A 26%	•	Vitamin C 31%	
Calcium 4%	•	Iron 18%	

Nutrition Grade B+

* Based on a 2000 calorie diet

Broccoli Cranberry Salad with Rice

```
Nutrition Facts
Serving Size 238 g
Amount Per Serving
Calories 457          Calories from Fat 193
                            % Daily Value*
Total Fat 21.4g                         33%
   Saturated Fat 4.0g                   20%
   Trans Fat 0.0g
Cholesterol 0mg                          0%
Sodium 15mg                              1%
Potassium 778mg                         22%
Total Carbohydrates 58.5g               19%
   Dietary Fiber 11.3g                  45%
   Sugars 8.3g
Protein 11.4g
Vitamin A 12%        •      Vitamin C 114%
Calcium 11%          •            Iron 15%
Nutrition Grade A
* Based on a 2000 calorie diet
```

Serves – 4

Cooks In- 20 minutes

Preparation time - 10 min

Difficulty- Easy

Ingredients

- Avocado -1 piece , Sliced
- Cranberries – ½ cup
- Garlic Cloves -3 piece , Crushed
- Almonds - ¾ cup
- Brown Rice – 1 cup
- Coconut oil – 1 Teaspoon
- Peas – 1 cup
- Broccoli – 1 piece
- Large Orange – 1 piece

Method

1. Take a bowl, chop the broccoli and steam it for 4-5 minutes.

2. Cook the brown rice.

3. In a frying pan add a teaspoon of coconut oil and heat it over medium heat.

4. Add broccoli, peas and garlic and cook it for 3-4 minutes.

5. In a serving dish place the rice.

6. Top it with broccoli, sprinkle almond and cranberries and avocado.

7. Mix lemon juice, pinch of salt and pepper and pour onto the rice.

8. Serve it warm...

3 Gluten Free – Dinner Recipes

Hot and Spicy Shrimp Curry

Serves – 4
Cooks In- 55 minutes
Preparation time - 5 min
Difficulty- Easy

Ingredients

- Shrimp – 450 grams
- Tomato Puree – 350 grams
- Olive Oil – 1 tablespoon
- Large Onions – 1 piece , Chopped
- Salt – 1 teaspoon
- Ground Pepper – ¼ teaspoon
- Garlic cloves – 2 Piece , Minced
- Green Capsicum – ½ piece , chopped
- Shrimp stock – 1 cup
- Soya sauce – 2 Teaspoon
- Lemon Juice – ¼ teaspoon
- Sugar – ¼ Teaspoon
- Fish sauce – 1/8 teaspoon
- Hot sauce – 1/8 teaspoon
- Red chili pepper powder – ½ Teaspoon

- Stalks celery – 1 piece , Chopped

Method

1. Take an oven-proof Skillet, heat it over medium heat.
2. Add olive oil, garlic, celery onions, and capsicum and cook it for 4-5 minutes until it is tender.
3. Add red chili pepper, pinch of salt and pepper powder and stir it.
4. Now add tomato puree, stock, soya sauce, lemon juice, fish sauce, hot sauce.
5. Simmer it for 30-35 minutes.
6. Add shrimps to the mixture and cook for another 5-6 minutes until its pink.
7. Serve and Enjoy it.

Nutrition Facts

Serving Size 318 g

Amount Per Serving	
Calories 232	Calories from Fat 56
	% Daily Value*
Total Fat 6.2g	10%
Saturated Fat 1.2g	6%
Trans Fat 0.0g	
Cholesterol 237mg	79%
Sodium 1149mg	48%
Potassium 770mg	22%
Total Carbohydrates 15.1g	5%
Dietary Fiber 2.8g	11%
Sugars 6.6g	
Protein 29.3g	
Vitamin A 20% •	Vitamin C 40%
Calcium 14% •	Iron 13%

Nutrition Grade A

* Based on a 2000 calorie diet

Pork Chops with Cinnamon Apple

Serves – 2
Cooks In- 55 minutes
Preparation time - 10 min
Difficulty- Easy

Ingredients

- Garlic powder - ½ teaspoon
- Salt – ¼ teaspoon
- Butter – 1 tablespoon
- Ground Pepper – ½ Teaspoon
- Dijon mustard – 4 Tablespoon
- Virgin Olive Oil – 4 tablespoon
- Pork Loin Chops – 4 piece , Boneless and sliced thin
- Ground Cinnamon – ½ teaspoon
- Brown sugar – 1 ½ tablespoon
- Apple – 2 Medium ,Thinly sliced

Method

1. Pre Heat oven to 350 degree F.
2. Take a bowl mix pepper, garlic powder, salt.
3. Prepare a baking sheet with parchment pour, grease it with oil.

4. Pour the mustard mixture over the pork chops.
5. Place the baking sheet into the oven for 40-45 minutes.
6. In a bowl, mix cinnamon, brown sugar and apple.
7. Take a frying pan and cook the apple with the mixture.
8. Flip side of pork chops occasionally.
9. Once chops are light pinkish on the center it's done.
10. Serve the chops with Apple. Dash it with honey if you want.

Nutrition Facts

Serving Size 420 g

Amount Per Serving

Calories 949	Calories from Fat 676
	% Daily Value*
Total Fat 75.1g	116%
Saturated Fat 22.6g	113%
Trans Fat 0.0g	
Cholesterol 153mg	51%
Sodium 802mg	33%
Potassium 816mg	23%
Total Carbohydrates 34.8g	12%
Dietary Fiber 6.0g	24%
Sugars 25.9g	
Protein 38.1g	

Vitamin A 4%	•	Vitamin C 26%
Calcium 8%	•	Iron 17%

Nutrition Grade B-

* Based on a 2000 calorie diet

Strawberries with Sautéed Chicken Salad

Serves – 2
Cooks In- 20 minutes
Preparation time - 10 min
Difficulty- Easy

Ingredients

- Olive oil – 4 tablespoon
- Salt – ½ teaspoon
- Ground Pepper – ¼ teaspoon
- Boneless Chicken Breast – 10 oz.
- Blueberries – 1 cup
- Strawberries – 1 cup ,Sliced
- Almond -4 pieces ,Toasted and sliced
- Yogurt – 3 oz.
- Mayonnaise - 1 ½ Tablespoon

Method

1. Take a non-sticky frying pan pour oil and cook the chicken for 5-6 minutes over medium heat. Flip side until chicken is cooked properly. Remove it from the pan. Slice it into cubes.
2. Take a bowl mix all the ingredients except the cooked chicken and almond.
3. Add the chicken and toss it gently so it's mixed properly with the mixture.

4. Refrigerate for 10 minutes.
5. Serve it and enjoy.

Nutrition Facts

Serving Size 374 g

Amount Per Serving	
Calories 662	Calories from Fat 399
	% Daily Value*
Total Fat 44.4g	68%
Saturated Fat 8.0g	40%
Trans Fat 0.0g	
Cholesterol 132mg	44%
Sodium 813mg	34%
Potassium 632mg	18%
Total Carbohydrates 22.3g	7%
Dietary Fiber 3.6g	14%
Sugars 14.5g	
Protein 45.1g	

Vitamin A 3%	•	Vitamin C 90%
Calcium 12%	•	Iron 18%

Nutrition Grade B-

* Based on a 2000 calorie diet

Superb Steaks with Mushroom Fries

Serves – 2
Cooks In- 20 minutes
Preparation time - 10 min
Difficulty- Easy

Ingredients

- Salt – ¼ Teaspoon
- Ground Pepper – ¼ teaspoon
- Baby Portobello Mushroom – 150 grams , Sliced
- 5-Spice Powder – Dash
- Ginger – ½ Tablespoon, Minced
- Olive Oil – 1 Tablespoon
- Strip Steak – ½ pound , Sliced small
- Coriander Leaves – ½ cup , Chopped
- Hoisin sauce – 2 ½ Tablespoon
- Green Onion - ½ bunch , Chopped

Method

1. Take a bowl and season the beef steak, salt, pepper, 5–Spice powder, and hoisin sauce.
2. Whisk it properly. Keep it aside for 10 minutes.

3. Pour 1 tablespoon Oil in to a large skillet and fry over medium heat, the meat for 3-5 minutes until the meat turns light brown. Remove meat from the skillet.
4. Pour rest of the oil in the skillet, add the mushroom and minced ginger and cook it for 5-8 minutes until the mushrooms are tender.
5. Add the meat and cook for another 10– 12 minutes.
6. Then add Coriander and green onion. Keep some for dressing.
7. Stir and cook for another 3-4 minutes.
8. Serve it and top it with left coriander and green onion.

Nutrition Facts

Serving Size 247 g

Amount Per Serving

Calories 360	Calories from Fat 123
	% Daily Value*
Total Fat 13.7g	21%
Saturated Fat 3.1g	16%
Cholesterol 103mg	34%
Sodium 675mg	28%
Potassium 752mg	21%
Total Carbohydrates 14.4g	5%
Dietary Fiber 2.3g	9%
Sugars 7.4g	
Protein 44.7g	
Vitamin A 10%	Vitamin C 14%
Calcium 3%	Iron 38%

Nutrition Grade A-

* Based on a 2000 calorie diet

Cheesy Chicken with Healthy Broccoli Rice

Serves – 2
Cooks In- 30 minutes
Preparation time - 25 min
Difficulty- Easy

Ingredients

- Boneless Chicken - 150 grams(¼ pound)
- Chicken Stock - ¾ cup
- Brown Rice – ¾ cups
- Flour – 2 Teaspoon
- Salt – ¼ Teaspoon
- Ground Pepper - ¼ Teaspoon
- Garlic Powder – ¼ Teaspoon
- Yogurt – 2 Tablespoon
- Broccoli Florets – 150 grams (¼ Pound), Chopped
- Olive Oil – ¼ Teaspoon
- Dijon Mustard -1 Tablespoon
- Cheese – 50 grams, Shredded
- Skim Milk – ¾ cup

Method

1. Take a large skillet with cover, pour chicken stock and boil it. Add rice and boil it again, reduce heat then add broccoli, cover it and cook for 4-5 minutes. Keep it aside.
2. In big pan pour oil heat it, add chicken, half salt, pepper and garlic powder, fry chicken for 5-6 minutes until it is light brown. Take it out in a plate
3. Now we will make the sauce, take a bowl add flour and half skim milk, whisk it.
4. Pour it into the pan and then add rest of the milk heat it, cook while stirring until its thick for 8-10 minutes.
5. Remove it from heat; add mustard, remaining salt, pepper, and garlic powder. Whisk the mixture properly and then add yogurt and some cheese. Stir it until it is smooth.
6. Now for the baking process, add chicken and rice to the sauce. Stir it gently so that everything is mixed properly.
7. Take a deep baking dish with parchment pour, grease it with oil.
8. Evenly place the chicken and rice mixture on the baking sheet, shred the remaining cheese on the top.
9. Bake it on a pre-heated oven for 25 minutes.
10. Serve it when it's warm. Enjoy...

Chicken and Mixed Vegetable Stew

```
                Nutrition Facts
Serving Size 455 g

Amount Per Serving
Calories 597              Calories from Fat 156
                                    % Daily Value*
Total Fat 17.4g                            27%
    Saturated Fat 7.5g                     37%
    Trans Fat 0.0g
Cholesterol 96mg                           32%
Sodium 973mg                               41%
Potassium 840mg                            24%
Total Carbohydrates 68.2g                  23%
    Dietary Fiber 4.8g                     19%
    Sugars 7.4g
Protein 40.2g
Vitamin A 19%        •        Vitamin C 114%
Calcium 40%          •             Iron 18%
Nutrition Grade A-
* Based on a 2000 calorie diet
```

Serves – 4

Cooks In- 30 minutes

Preparation time - 30 min

Difficulty- Easy

Ingredients

- Tomato Paste – ¼ can
- Tomato – 2 Piece , Medium ,Diced
- Olive oil – ½ Tablespoon
- Chicken Breast – ¼ pound , Diced
- Capsicum – ½ piece , Diced
- Onion – ¼ cup, Diced
- Garlic Clove – 2 piece , Chopped
- Carrots – 1 piece , Diced
- Salt – ¼ Tablespoon

- Ground Pepper – ¼ Teaspoon
- Zucchini – 1 piece , Small and Diced
- Fresh Basil - ¼ cup , chopped
- Mushroom – ¼ cup , Diced
- Cheese – Grated , To Dress
- Baby spinach – 1 Handful , OPTIONAL

Method

1. Take a large Dutch oven or a crock pot.
2. Add diced chicken, vegetables and tomato and sauce. Except the cheese.
3. Cook for 3-4 hours (HIGH) or 6-8 hours (LOW), stirring occasionally for every 30 minutes.
4. Once it is ready, serve it with grated cheese.

Nutrition Facts

Serving Size 177 g

Amount Per Serving	
Calories 123	Calories from Fat 43
	% Daily Value*
Total Fat 4.7g	7%
Saturated Fat 1.4g	7%
Trans Fat 0.0g	
Cholesterol 30mg	10%
Sodium 541mg	23%
Potassium 566mg	16%
Total Carbohydrates 9.0g	3%
Dietary Fiber 2.4g	10%
Sugars 4.6g	
Protein 12.7g	
Vitamin A 89%	Vitamin C 53%
Calcium 8%	Iron 9%

Nutrition Grade A

* Based on a 2000 calorie diet

Pineapple Roasted Pork

Serves – 2
Cooks In- 20 minutes
Preparation time - 15 min
Difficulty- Easy

Ingredients

- Olive oil – 1 Tablespoon
- Salt – ¼ Teaspoon
- Ground Pepper - ¼ Teaspoon
- Pork Loin (Rib) – 12 oz.
- Onion – ¼ cup , Chopped
- Brown Sugar – ½ Tablespoon
- Apple cider Vinegar – ½ Tablespoon
- Pineapple - 5 oz. ,Crushed
- Cinnamon – Pinch ,Grounded
- Ginger – Pinch , Grounded

Method

1. Preheat the oven to 425 degree F.
2. Take the pork, add pepper and salt. Rub it properly.
3. Take the skillet & pour oil, heat it over medium heat.
4. Place the meat and cook it by flipping for 2-3 minutes until all sides are light brown.

5. Then bake it in the oven for 20 – 25 minutes until they are slightly pinkish in colour.
6. While meat is baking, take a saucepan, add onion & cook it for 4-5 minutes over medium-heat, until it is light brown.
7. Add sugar, pineapple, vinegar, cinnamon, and ginger to the saucepan. Bring it to boil.
8. Reduce heat and simmer for 15 minutes and stir it occasionally until it is thick like syrup.
9. Serve it with the warm pork loin.

Nutrition Facts

Serving Size 270 g

Amount Per Serving	
Calories 524	Calories from Fat 277

	% Daily Value*
Total Fat 30.8g	47%
Saturated Fat 9.9g	50%
Trans Fat 0.0g	
Cholesterol 136mg	45%
Sodium 399mg	17%
Potassium 831mg	24%
Total Carbohydrates 13.4g	4%
Dietary Fiber 1.6g	6%
Sugars 9.8g	
Protein 47.1g	

Vitamin A 1%	•	Vitamin C 60%
Calcium 5%	•	Iron 10%

Nutrition Grade B

* Based on a 2000 calorie diet

Juicy Lamb Kebabs with Veggies

Serves – 2
Cooks In- 15 minutes
Preparation time - 40 min
Difficulty- Easy

Ingredients

- Olive oil – 2 Tablespoon
- Salt – ½ Teaspoon
- Ground Pepper - ¼ teaspoon
- Chili powder – ¼ Teaspoon
- Boneless Leg of Lamb – ¼ pound ,Chopped
- Onion – 4 small pieces, Whole
- Tomato – 4 Small pieces, Whole
- Garlic cloves – 1 piece ,chopped
- Garlic paste – ¼ Tablespoon
- Ginger paste – ¼ Tablespoon
- Lemon – ½ piece
- Small Carrot – 1 piece , Sliced
- Lettuce – Chopped

Method

1. Take a bowl, mix salt and pepper and half ginger-garlic paste.

2. Add lamb, carrot, tomatoes and onions, squeeze some lemon juice, toss it and keep it for 30 minutes to marinate.
3. Take metal skewers; thread marinated lamb pieces, carrots, tomatoes and onion one by one. Keep distance between them.
4. On barbecue grill keep the skewers and heat over medium heat for 4-5 minutes until lamb are light brown in colour each side, and vegetables are tender.
5. Brush oil and leftover mixture from the bowl, occasionally while rotating the skewer.
6. Lamb kebabs are ready. Segregate lamb and vegetables.
7. Serve on a plate, place lettuce, lamb and the vegetable. Sprinkle salt, pepper and lemon juice as per your taste.
8. You can also use sliced capsicum along with vegetables.

Nutrition Facts

Serving Size 539 g

Amount Per Serving	
Calories 371	Calories from Fat 171
	% Daily Value*
Total Fat 19.0g	29%
Saturated Fat 3.6g	18%
Trans Fat 0.0g	
Cholesterol 51mg	17%
Sodium 665mg	28%
Potassium 1101mg	31%
Total Carbohydrates 33.5g	11%
Dietary Fiber 8.3g	33%
Sugars 15.9g	
Protein 20.7g	
Vitamin A 116%	Vitamin C 82%
Calcium 10%	Iron 19%

Nutrition Grade A
* Based on a 2000 calorie diet

Juicy Salmon with Lemony Sweet Potatoes

Serves – 2
Cooks In- 15 minutes
Preparation time - 15 min
Difficulty- Easy

Ingredients

- Olive oil – 2 Tablespoon
- Skinless Salmon Fillet – 2 Piece , Centre Cut
- Sweet potatoes - ½ pound
- Salt – ¼ Teaspoon
- Ground pepper – ¼ teaspoon
- Lemon – ½ Piece
- Capers – 1 tablespoon
- Chili powder – ¼ teaspoon
- White Grape juice – ½ cup
- Parsley – ¼ cup , Chopped

Method

1. In a skillet pour some oil; add salmon sprinkled with pinch of chili powder salt and pepper.
2. Cook it for 10 minutes; flip it occasionally until it is soft. Transfer it to a plate.
3. In a micro oven place a bowl with mixed potatoes, salt, pepper and water.

4. Cover it and cook it for 7-8 minutes until potatoes are tender.
5. Take the skillet pour white grape juice, caper and boil it for 2-3 minutes. Then remove the skillet from heat.
6. Squeeze Lemon juice and parsley and stir it. Your sauce is ready
7. On a plate place potatoes then salmon fillets.
8. Pour sauce on to the fillets by using spoon.
9. Serve your Salmon Fillets and enjoy.

Nutrition Facts		
Serving Size 391 g		
Amount Per Serving		
Calories 522		Calories from Fat 229
		% Daily Value*
Total Fat 25.4g		39%
Saturated Fat 3.6g		18%
Trans Fat 0.0g		
Cholesterol 78mg		26%
Sodium 515mg		21%
Potassium 1776mg		51%
Total Carbohydrates 39.3g		13%
Dietary Fiber 5.6g		22%
Sugars 6.5g		
Protein 37.1g		
Vitamin A 21%	•	Vitamin C 98%
Calcium 10%	•	Iron 14%
Nutrition Grade B		
* Based on a 2000 calorie diet		

Cheese Lasagna with Beef Sauce

Serves – 2
Cooks In- 15 minutes
Preparation time - 15 min
Difficulty- Easy

Ingredients

- Quinoa - ¼ cup
- Cheese
- Water - ¼ cup
- Onion Medium – ¼ piece, Chopped
- Mushroom – 2 Can (4oz.)
- Ground Beef – ¼ pound
- Tomato sauce – 8 oz.
- Oregano – ¼ Tablespoon
- Garlic Clove – 1 Piece
- Lasagna noodles – 1 pound box
- Olive oil

Method

1. Preheat oven at 375 degree F.
2. In a frying pan over medium heat put 1 tablespoon oil, onion and garlic.
3. Then add beef and fry until it is brown.
4. Place mushroom, oregano, tomato sauce, quinoa and water. Stir it, bring it to boil,
5. Reduce heat then simmer for 10-12 minutes.
6. Prepare a baking dish

7. Place a layer of beef sauce, then lasagna noodles followed by a layer of sauce and noodle.
8. Add a thin layer of cheese, place a layer of noodles and then a layer of sauce.
9. Top it with a thick layer of grated cheese (you can use mozzarella and parmesan cheese).
10. Cover the baking dish and bake for 45 minutes.
11. Uncover it and bake for another 15 minutes.
12. Serve it and enjoy.

Nutrition Facts

Serving Size 600 g

Amount Per Serving

Calories 964	Calories from Fat 157
	% Daily Value*
Total Fat 17.4g	27%
Saturated Fat 3.3g	16%
Cholesterol 130mg	43%
Sodium 664mg	28%
Potassium 1160mg	33%
Total Carbohydrates 150.8g	50%
Dietary Fiber 5.0g	20%
Sugars 7.6g	
Protein 53.3g	

Vitamin A 9%	•	Vitamin C 22%
Calcium 7%	•	Iron 93%

Nutrition Grade B+

* Based on a 2000 calorie diet

4 Gluten-Free Soups Recipes

Super Delicious Spinach Soup

Serves – 4-6
Cooks In- 15 minutes
Preparation time - 15 min
Difficulty- Easy

Ingredients

- Salt – ¼ Tablespoon
- Cooking oil – 1 Tablespoon
- Ground Pepper – ¼ Teaspoon
- Garlic clove – 2 piece, Crushed
- Water – 2 cup
- Vegetable Broth – 6 cup
- Large Carrots – 3 piece , Diced
- Large Onion - 1 piece, Diced
- Spinach – 2 bunch , Chopped
- Tomato Can – 14 oz., Diced
- Celery Stalks – 2 piece, Diced
- Green Lentils – 2 cups, Rinsed

Method

1. Take a large skillet, on medium heat, pour oil.

2. Add chopped onion and garlic and fry until it softens.
3. Then add celery and carrots, fry for another 4-5 minutes and then add lentils and fry for 4-5 minutes.
4. Finally add salt, pepper, vegetable broth and tomatoes. Boil it for ½ hour, covered.
5. Remove from heat, add spinach.
6. Serve it warm.
7. You can dress it with grated cheese on top if you want.

Nutrition Facts

Serving Size 792 g

Amount Per Serving

Calories 488	Calories from Fat 61
	% Daily Value*
Total Fat 6.8g	10%
Saturated Fat 1.3g	6%
Trans Fat 0.0g	
Cholesterol 0mg	0%
Sodium 1653mg	69%
Potassium 1790mg	51%
Total Carbohydrates 73.0g	24%
Dietary Fiber 33.1g	132%
Sugars 10.0g	
Protein 34.3g	

Vitamin A 222%	•	Vitamin C 47%
Calcium 13%	•	Iron 50%

Nutrition Grade A

* Based on a 2000 calorie diet

Gingery Soupy Chicken Noodles

Serves – 6
Cooks In- 15 minutes
Preparation time - 15 min
Difficulty- Easy

Ingredients

- Salt – ¼ Tablespoon
- Ground Pepper – ¼ Teaspoon
- Garlic clove – 6 piece, Crushed
- Chicken Broth – 10 cup
- Large Carrots – 2 piece , Diced
- Chicken Breast - 1 Lbs., Cooked
- Ginger – 3 Tablespoon, Minced
- Fresh Dill – 2 Tablespoon , Chopped
- Lemon Juice – 1 Tablespoon
- Celery Stalks – 1 piece, Diced
- Gluten free Egg noodles – 4 oz.

Method

1. In a large skillet, pour chicken broth and bring it to boil.
2. Add ginger, garlic, carrots and celery.

3. Cook over medium heat, for 20-25 minutes, until vegetables soften.
4. Then add lemon juice, dill, noodles and chicken, reduce heat and simmer for 8-10 minutes until the noodles are tender. Stir it occasionally.
5. Serve it in noodle bowl.

Nutrition Facts

Serving Size 531 g

Amount Per Serving	
Calories 242	Calories from Fat 50
	% Daily Value*
Total Fat 5.6g	9%
Saturated Fat 0.8g	4%
Trans Fat 0.0g	
Cholesterol 70mg	23%
Sodium 1674mg	70%
Potassium 714mg	20%
Total Carbohydrates 12.3g	4%
Dietary Fiber 1.4g	6%
Sugars 2.6g	
Protein 34.1g	
Vitamin A 82%	• Vitamin C 7%
Calcium 7%	• Iron 16%

Nutrition Grade A
* Based on a 2000 calorie diet

Tomatina Basil Soup

Serves – 4
Cooks In- 15 minutes
Preparation time - 15 min
Difficulty- Easy

Ingredients

- Salt – ¼ teaspoon
- Ground Pepper – ¼ teaspoon
- Basil – ¾ cup
- Tomatoes – 28 oz., Chopped
- Olive oil – 2 Tablespoon
- Vegetable broth – 2 cups
- Balsamic vinegar – ½ tablespoon
- Cream or Cheese - optional
- Onion – 1 ½ cups, Chopped
- Garlic cloves – 3 piece, 1 piece Halved and 2 piece chopped
- Sugar – ½ tablespoon.

Method

1. In a skillet with cover, heat oil over medium heat.
2. Add onion and fry for 6-7 minutes until it is translucent.

3. Add sugar, salt, pepper, vinegar and garlic, fry for another 2-3 minutes.
4. Place tomatoes into the mixture and simmer it for 10 minutes while stirring.
5. Then add vegetable broth and simmer it again for 5 minutes.
6. Your soup is ready by now. Add salt and pepper as per you taste.
7. Top it with some cream or cheese if you like.
8. Serve it hot.

Nutrition Facts

Serving Size 381 g

Amount Per Serving	
Calories 147	Calories from Fat 76
	% Daily Value*
Total Fat 8.5g	13%
Saturated Fat 1.5g	7%
Trans Fat 0.0g	
Cholesterol 1mg	0%
Sodium 543mg	23%
Potassium 664mg	19%
Total Carbohydrates 14.9g	5%
Dietary Fiber 3.4g	14%
Sugars 9.1g	
Protein 5.0g	

Vitamin A 38%	•	Vitamin C 53%
Calcium 5%	•	Iron 6%

Nutrition Grade A-

* Based on a 2000 calorie diet

Zesty Zucchini Soup

Serves – 2
Cooks In- 30 minutes
Preparation time - 35 min
Difficulty- Easy

Ingredients

- Salt – ½ teaspoon
- Ground Pepper – ¼ teaspoon
- Small Zucchini – 1 Piece ,Sliced
- Vegetable broth – 2 cups
- Baby Spinach leaves – ¾ cup.
- Cauliflower Florets – 1 ¼ pound
- Olive Oil – 1 Tablespoon
- Sweet Potatoes – ½ Pound, Peeled and Chopped
- Chili Powder – ¼ Teaspoon
- Large Onion – 1 Piece, Chopped

Method

1. Take a large saucepan heat over medium heat, pour 1 tablespoon of oil.
2. Fry onion for 2-3 minutes until it is translucent.
3. Add Zucchini, potatoes and cauliflower, add salt, pepper, and pinch of chili powder.
4. Cook for 2-3 minutes, stirring.
5. Add vegetable broth, bring to boil.

6. Reduce heat and simmer for 25-30 minutes, until vegetables are tender. Add spinach.
7. Pour the mixture into blender and blend it until soup is smooth.
8. Top it with cream and serve it when warm.

Nutrition Facts

Serving Size 792 g

Amount Per Serving	
Calories 347	Calories from Fat 82

	% Daily Value*
Total Fat 9.1g	14%
Saturated Fat 1.5g	8%
Trans Fat 0.0g	
Cholesterol 0mg	0%
Sodium 1461mg	61%
Potassium 2327mg	66%
Total Carbohydrates 57.3g	19%
Dietary Fiber 14.4g	58%
Sugars 12.3g	
Protein 14.1g	

Vitamin A 29%	•	Vitamin C 283%	
Calcium 13%	•	Iron 18%	

Nutrition Grade A

* Based on a 2000 calorie diet

Kale Soup with Chicken Sausages

Serves – 4
Cooks In- 15 minutes
Preparation time - 15 min
Difficulty- Easy

Ingredients

- Salt – ¼ teaspoon
- Ground Pepper – ¼ teaspoon
- Spicy Chicken Sausage – ¾ pound
- Olive oil – 2 Tablespoon
- Chicken broth – 6 cups
- Kale – 2 Bunch, Stemmed and chopped
- Baked Potatoes – 3 medium, Sliced
- Cream – ½ cup
- Onion – 1 ½ cups, Chopped
- Garlic cloves – 3 piece, Chopped
- Nutmeg – ¼ teaspoon.

Method

1. Take a large skillet over medium heat, heat it and add sausage, cook it until it is fully brown, stirring occasionally. Remove the sausage in to a plate. Lower the heat

2. Then add oil to the pan and sauté onion and garlic for 3- 5 minutes, until it is translucent.
3. Add salt and pepper, sauté again until the onions have caramelized.
4. Then add kale, handful of kale at a time. Cook for 3 minutes until kale is bright green.
5. Add in cooked sausage and potatoes.
6. Finally add chicken broth, bring it to boil .Simmer it for 5-8 minutes until potatoes softens.
7. Taste it, adjust salt and pepper as per your taste.
8. Top it with cream and serve it.

Nutrition Facts

Serving Size 678 g

Amount Per Serving

Calories 448	Calories from Fat 183
	% Daily Value*
Total Fat 20.3g	31%
Saturated Fat 5.7g	28%
Trans Fat 0.0g	
Cholesterol 6mg	2%
Sodium 1659mg	69%
Potassium 1129mg	32%
Total Carbohydrates 42.2g	14%
Dietary Fiber 5.2g	21%
Sugars 5.1g	
Protein 22.8g	

Vitamin A 40%	•	Vitamin C 84%
Calcium 7%	•	Iron 13%

Nutrition Grade B-

* Based on a 2000 calorie diet

Turkey Soup with Tortilla

Serves – 6
Cooks In - 25 minutes
Preparation time - 40 min
Difficulty - Easy

Ingredients

- Salt – 2 ¼ Tablespoon
- Olive oil – 1 Tablespoon
- Ground Pepper – ¼ Teaspoon
- Oregano – ½ Teaspoon , Dried
- Garlic clove – 2 piece, Crushed
- Turkey Breast – 1 ½ Pound , Cooked and Boneless
- Green Onion – 2 Piece , Chopped
- Medium Onion – 1 Piece , Chopped finely
- Large Carrots – 1 Piece , Chopped finely
- Green Chili Pepper – 1 Piece , Sliced into Rings
- Chicken Broth – 6 cup
- Lime – 1 Piece , Wedges
- Fresh Coriander big Bunch - 1 piece, Chopped
- Ground Coriander – ½ Teaspoon
- Avocado – ½ Piece, Chopped and Peeled
- Ground Cumin – ½ Teaspoon
- Corn Tortillas – 2 piece

Method

1. Preheat the oven at 375 degree F.
2. Take a large Pot heat it over medium heat, add oil
3. Add carrot and onion and fry for 10-12 minutes, until its translucent, stir it occasionally.
4. Add salt, pepper, garlic, half cumin, oregano, and coriander powder, and stir in fresh coriander stem(keep the leaves for topping).Cook for 2 minutes over medium heat and then pour broth, bring it to boil. Reduce the heat and simmer for 20 minutes. Stir it occasionally.
5. Now we will make tortilla strips.
6. Take a bowl, cut corn Tortilla into ½ - inch strips. Add to the bowl, pour same oil season it, sprinkle pepper, salt, coriander, cumin powder, oregano, red chili powder. Toss it properly until seasoning coats on the tortilla evenly.
7. Take a baking sheet with parchment pour, grease it with some oil and then place the Tortilla strips and bake it for 20 minutes until it's crispy. Halfway through toss it so that it is evenly baked.
8. Now take a strainer, pour the soup. Retain the liquid in to a bowl. Solids are to be discarded.
9. Add turkey breast in to the soup and cook for 5-10 minutes.

10. Now serve the soup, top it with coriander leaves, avocado, green chili pepper, green onion, and tortilla strips to each bowl of soup.

11. ENJOY!

Shrimpy Seafood Soup

Nutrition Facts

Nutrition Facts	
Serving Size 436 g	
Amount Per Serving	
Calories 248	Calories from Fat 83
	% Daily Value*
Total Fat 9.2g	14%
Saturated Fat 1.8g	9%
Trans Fat 0.0g	
Cholesterol 49mg	16%
Sodium 4549mg	190%
Potassium 783mg	22%
Total Carbohydrates 15.2g	5%
Dietary Fiber 3.5g	14%
Sugars 6.5g	
Protein 25.7g	
Vitamin A 54%	Vitamin C 25%
Calcium 5%	Iron 16%
Nutrition Grade A	
* Based on a 2000 calorie diet	

Serves – 4
Cooks In- 20 minutes
Preparation time - 15 min
Difficulty- Easy

Ingredients

- Salt – 2 Tablespoon
- Olive oil – 1 Tablespoon
- Ground Pepper – ¼ Teaspoon
- Red Capsicum – 1 Piece , Diced and Seeded
- Oregano – ½ Teaspoon , Dried

- Garlic clove – 3 piece, Crushed
- White Fish – 1 ¼ Pound , Cut in to 1 inch size (such as plaice, halibut, cod, and haddock)
- Dry White Wine – ½ cup
- Medium Onion – 1 Piece , Chopped finely
- Large Carrot – 1 Piece , Chopped finely
- Chili Flakes – ¼ Teaspoon
- Vegetable Broth – 4 cup
- Medium Shrimp - ½ Pound, Shelled
- Tomatoes - 1 can (28 oz.), With juices
- Parsley – ½ cup ,Chopped
- Capers- 2 Tablespoon

Method

1. Take a large saucepan heat it over medium heat, pour olive oil.
2. Add carrot, capsicum, onion, garlic, cook for 8-9 minutes until it translucent (tender). Stir it occasionally.
3. Add chili flakes and oregano and cook for 2 minutes.
4. Then add parsley and white wine, cook for 1 minute.
5. Add vegetable broth and tomatoes with juices, bring it to boil. Reduce heat and simmer for 5 minutes. Keep stirring
6. Then add white fish to the soup and cook for 4-5 minutes. Stir occasionally.

7. Finally add shrimp and simmer for another 3-4 minutes. Remove from heat.
8. Add capers, stir it add salt and pepper as per your taste.
9. Serve it and Enjoy!

Creamy Ham Shank Soup with Lentil

Nutrition Facts

Serving Size 752 g

Amount Per Serving	
Calories 536	Calories from Fat 196
	% Daily Value*
Total Fat 21.8g	33%
Saturated Fat 1.0g	5%
Trans Fat 0.0g	
Cholesterol 111mg	37%
Sodium 4538mg	189%
Potassium 902mg	26%
Total Carbohydrates 51.9g	17%
Dietary Fiber 7.0g	28%
Sugars 9.0g	
Protein 29.9g	

Vitamin A 109%	•	Vitamin C 99%	
Calcium 8%	•	Iron 22%	

Nutrition Grade C+
* Based on a 2000 calorie diet

Serves – 6
Cooks in- 3 Hours
Preparation time - 15 min
Difficulty- Easy

Ingredients

- Ham Shank – 1 piece
- Butter – 3 Tablespoon
- Cream – 4 oz. Fluid
- Curry Powder – 1 Teaspoon
- Lentils – 20 oz., Rinsed
- Large Onion – 1 Piece , Chopped

- Garlic Cloves – 2 Piece, Chopped
- Medium Carrots – 2 Piece, Chopped
- Celery – 3 sticks, Chopped
- Nutmeg – ¼ Teaspoon

Method

1. Take a large pot, put ham sank, pour water and bring it to boil then simmer for 2 hours. Until meat and bone are segregated.
2. Take a large frying pan, add butter and then fry onion, celery, and carrots for 15-20 minutes until it is translucent. Stir it occasionally
3. Add garlic to the frying pan and cook for another 2 minutes.
4. Now remove ham from the pot and reserve the water in a bowl.
5. Take the frying pan, heat it over medium heat, add earlier cooked vegetables, along with lentils and remaining ingredients except the cream and then add ham, toss it and sauté for 2- 3 minutes.
6. Use a strainer to remove the layer of impurities. Add rest of water to the pot.
7. Bring the mixture to boil, reduce the heat and simmer it or 25-30 minutes until lentils are tender and cooked.
8. Blend the mixture to get a smooth texture.
9. Set it aside to cool
10. Top it with cream and serve.

Soupy Chicken Pesto Meatballs with Rice

```
Nutrition Facts
Serving Size 855 g
Amount Per Serving
Calories 993              Calories from Fat 346
                                    % Daily Value*
Total Fat 38.4g                            59%
   Saturated Fat 8.7g                      44%
   Trans Fat 0.0g
Cholesterol 155mg                          52%
Sodium 5442mg                             227%
Potassium 1929mg                           55%
Total Carbohydrates 87.6g                  29%
   Dietary Fiber 11.2g                     45%
   Sugars 7.3g
Protein 67.4g
Vitamin A 68%         •       Vitamin C 5%
Calcium 38%           •           Iron 63%
Nutrition Grade C+
* Based on a 2000 calorie diet
```

Serves – 4
Cooks In- 15 minutes
Preparation time - 15 min
Difficulty- Easy

Ingredients

- Salt – 2 Tablespoon
- Olive oil – 3 Tablespoon
- Ground Pepper – ¼ Teaspoon
- Cooked Rice – 1 cup
- Bread Crumbs – 2 tablespoon
- Egg – 1 Piece
- Fresh Pesto – ½ cup
- Parmesan Cheese – ½ cup
- Ground Chicken – 1 Pound
- Dry White Wine – ½ cup
- Medium Onion – 1 Piece , Chopped finely

- Large Carrot – 1 Piece , Chopped finely
- Celery – 2 Sticks, Chopped finely
- Chicken Broth – 8 cup
- Flour – 3 Tablespoon
- White Beans – 8 oz.

Method

1. Take a mixing bowl; add fresh pesto, chicken and bread crumbs. Toss it properly.
2. Make meatballs by rolling between your palms (1 inch size).
3. In a stock pot add 2 tablespoon oil, heat it over medium heat, brown meatballs .Keep it aside.
4. Pour rest of oil to the pot, add carrots and onions and fry it for 2-3 minutes until it is soft and tender.
5. Then add celery and cook for 3 minutes on medium heat.
6. Stir in flour into the pot and cook for another 2-3 minute. Keep stirring it to avoid any lump formation.
7. Add white wine and then chicken broth, while stirring.
8. Now add beans and cooked rice, cook for 5 minutes, stir is properly.
9. A thick soup will be ready by now.
10. Finally add meatballs cooked earlier, simmer for 10-15 minutes.
11. Your meatball soup is ready. Taste it and add salt and pepper as per taste.

12. Serve it hot. Enjoy!

Delicious Beef Beans Soup

Serves – 4
Cooks In- 15 minutes
Preparation time - 15 min
Difficulty- Easy

Ingredients

- Salt – 2 Tablespoon
- Olive oil – 3 Tablespoon
- Ground Pepper – ¼ Teaspoon
- Beef Stew Meat- 1 pound, Chopped into 2 Inch size
- Medium Onion – 1 Piece , Chopped finely
- Large Carrot – 2 Piece , Chopped finely
- Bean soup Mix – ½ packet
- Celery – 2 Sticks, Chopped finely
- Vegetable Broth – 8 cup
- Tomato sauce – ½ can (15 oz.)
- Fresh Parsley ,Chopped finely
- Bay leaves – 1

Method

1. In a stock pot add 2 tablespoon oil, heat it over medium heat, brown beef stew. Keep it aside.

2. Pour rest of oil to the pot, add carrots and onions and celery fry it for 2-3 minutes until it is soft and tender. Stir it occasionally.
3. Then add vegetable broth, while stirring.
4. Now add beans, cook for 5 minutes, stir is properly.
5. Add the meat, tomato sauce and bay leaves, bring it to boil, lower the heat, simmer for 1 -1 ½ hours until beans and beef are tender. Keep stirring
6. Remove from heat. Top it with chopped parsley. Taste it and add salt and pepper as per taste.
7. Serve it hot. Enjoy!

Nutrition Facts

Serving Size 810 g

Amount Per Serving

Calories 469	Calories from Fat 189
	% Daily Value*
Total Fat 21.0g	32%
Saturated Fat 5.0g	25%
Trans Fat 0.0g	
Cholesterol 101mg	34%
Sodium 5804mg	242%
Potassium 1568mg	45%
Total Carbohydrates 21.6g	7%
Dietary Fiber 5.2g	21%
Sugars 9.5g	
Protein 48.4g	

Vitamin A 149%	•	Vitamin C 45%
Calcium 10%	•	Iron 144%

Nutrition Grade A
* Based on a 2000 calorie diet

5 Gluten-Free Desserts Recipes

Vanilla Rice Pudding

Serves – 6
Cooks In- 30 minutes
Preparation time - 5 min
Difficulty- Easy

Ingredients

- Rice – ¼ cup ,Short Grain
- Milk – 1 ½ cup
- Vanilla extract – 1 Tablespoon
- Raisins – 1 tablespoon
- Salt – ¼ Teaspoon
- Granulated Sugar – 2 Tablespoon
- Cinnamon - ¼ Teaspoon
- Table cream – ½ cup

Method

1. Take a sauce pan with cover, heat it over medium heat, add rice, milk, salt, cinnamon and cream. Bring it to boil. Stir it occasionally.

2. Reduce heat and simmer it for 20-25 minutes, keep stirring. Add raisins.
3. Cover the saucepan and simmer for another 5 minutes until rice is soft and tender.
4. Finally stir in vanilla extract.
5. Serve it warm or you can refrigerate and serve it cold.

Nutrition Facts

Serving Size 97 g

Amount Per Serving

Calories 124	Calories from Fat 47
	% Daily Value*
Total Fat 5.2g	8%
Saturated Fat 3.2g	16%
Trans Fat 0.0g	
Cholesterol 18mg	6%
Sodium 134mg	6%
Potassium 83mg	2%
Total Carbohydrates 15.4g	5%
Sugars 8.0g	
Protein 3.1g	

Vitamin A 3%	•	Vitamin C 0%
Calcium 10%	•	Iron 2%

Nutrition Grade D+

* Based on a 2000 calorie diet

Gluten Free Chocolate Cake

Yield – 8 Inch
Difficulty- Easy

Ingredients

- Large Egg – 3 piece
- Unsalted Butter – ½ cup
- Chocolate – 4 Oz., Bittersweet
- Cocoa Powder – ½ cup, Unsweetened
- Sugar – ¾ cup

Method

1. Preheat oven to 375 degree F.
2. Prepare an 8 inch round baking pan with parchment paper (either butter or wax paper).
3. Take chocolates and chop it into small pieces.
4. Now take saucepan pour 1-2 cup water and bring it to boil, reduce heat and simmer.
5. Place a metal bowl over the saucepan with simmering water.
6. Add chopped chocolate with butter, after sometime it starts melting. Stir it until the mixture is smooth.
7. Remove the bowl from the saucepan.

8. Add sugar to the chocolate mixture and whisk it.

9. Now break eggs and add the liquid to the mixture, whisk it well.

10. Finally add cocoa powder to the mixture, whisk it properly until all the ingredients combine together and no bubbles are there. Batter is ready.

11. Pour the batter into the round baking pan.

12. Bake it into the preheated oven for 25 minutes. Peirce knife into middle of the cake if it comes out clean your cake it almost complete.

13. Remove it from the oven, cool it for 5 minutes.

14. Invert the cake and serve it on a plate.

Nutrition Facts

Serving Size 95 g

Amount Per Serving

Calories 382	Calories from Fat 220
	% Daily Value*
Total Fat 24.4g	38%
Saturated Fat 15.0g	75%
Cholesterol 138mg	46%
Sodium 160mg	7%
Potassium 288mg	8%
Total Carbohydrates 40.4g	13%
Dietary Fiber 2.8g	11%
Sugars 35.1g	
Protein 6.1g	

Vitamin A 13%	•	Vitamin C 0%
Calcium 6%	•	Iron 11%

Nutrition Grade C

* Based on a 2000 calorie diet

Poached Pears with Maple Syrup

Serves – 3
Cooks In- 35 minutes
Preparation time - 15 min
Difficulty- Easy

Ingredients

- Water – 2 cup
- Ripe Pear – 3 Piece
- Plain Yogurt – ½ cup
- Apple juice – ½ cup
- Clove – 4 Piece, Whole
- Maple Syrup – ½ cup
- Cinnamon Stick – ½ piece

Method

1. Take a large saucepan; pour water, cinnamon stick, cloves, apple juice and maple syrup. Bring it to boil.
2. Now take a pear, peel it leaving the stem intact. See to it that it sits on a plate, otherwise trim bottom to level. Repeat the procedure for the rest of the pears.
3. Add all pears into the maple syrup mixture. Bring it to boil.

4. Reduce the heat and simmer for 25 minutes until tip of knife is easily pierced.
5. Using slotted spoon transfer all the pears to individual plates. Remove solids from the syrup you can use strainer to do so.
6. Pour the syrup again into the saucepan and boil it for 15-20 minutes until the syrup is reduced to thick syrup.
7. Finally pour the syrup over pears.
8. Serve it and Enjoy!

Nutrition Facts

Serving Size 434 g

Amount Per Serving	
Calories 272	Calories from Fat 10

	% Daily Value*
Total Fat 1.1g	2%
Saturated Fat 0.5g	3%
Trans Fat 0.0g	
Cholesterol 2mg	1%
Sodium 44mg	2%
Potassium 432mg	12%
Total Carbohydrates 65.4g	22%
Dietary Fiber 5.2g	21%
Sugars 52.2g	
Protein 2.9g	

Vitamin A 1%	•	Vitamin C 41%
Calcium 15%	•	Iron 7%

Nutrition Grade A
* Based on a 2000 calorie diet

Ricotta Mousse with Chocolate

Serves – 2
Difficulty- Easy

Ingredients

- Salt – ¼ Teaspoon
- Ricotta – 1 Cup
- Sugar – 1 ½ Tablespoon
- Chocolate powder – 4 Tablespoon , Unsweetened
- Large Egg – 1 piece, White

Method

1. Take a food processor or a blender.
2. Add chocolate powder and ricotta and blend it until smooth.
3. Take another bowl, add egg white, pinch of salt and sugar and cook it by whisking smoothly.(Place the bowl on top of simmering water pot).
4. Cook it for 3-4 minutes until sugar dissolves completely .
5. Using a whisker or electric mixture whisk it for 5- 6 minutes, until it is soft and firm.
6. Combine ricotta mixture and egg mixture properly.
7. Divide the mixture among bowls and refrigerate at least for 3 hours before serving.

8. Can top it with saved chocolate chips if you want.

Nutrition Facts	
Serving Size 243 g	
Amount Per Serving	
Calories 481	Calories from Fat 156
	% Daily Value*
Total Fat 17.3g	27%
Saturated Fat 6.9g	34%
Cholesterol 131mg	44%
Sodium 481mg	20%
Potassium 389mg	11%
Total Carbohydrates 51.6g	17%
Dietary Fiber 14.0g	56%
Sugars 9.6g	
Protein 27.3g	
Vitamin A 12%	Vitamin C 0%
Calcium 43%	Iron 38%
Nutrition Grade B-	
* Based on a 2000 calorie diet	

Coconut Cream with Berries

Nutrition Facts	
Serving Size 114 g	
Amount Per Serving	
Calories 225	Calories from Fat 113
	% Daily Value*
Total Fat 12.6g	19%
Saturated Fat 9.2g	46%
Trans Fat 0.0g	
Cholesterol 10mg	3%
Sodium 30mg	1%
Potassium 228mg	7%
Total Carbohydrates 25.7g	9%
Dietary Fiber 3.5g	14%
Sugars 19.7g	
Protein 2.9g	
Vitamin A 2% •	Vitamin C 30%
Calcium 7% •	Iron 7%
Nutrition Grade C+	
* Based on a 2000 calorie diet	

Serves – 2

Preparation time - 15 min

Difficulty- Easy

Ingredients

- Berries – ¼ pound ,
- Dark Chocolate
- Sugar – ¼ Tablespoon
- Cream – 4 Tablespoon
- Lime Juice – ¼ Tablespoon
- Coconut Cream – 2 Tablespoon

Method

1. Add heavy cream and coconut cream in to a electric mixture, whisk until soft peak form.
2. In a bowl mix berries, lime juice and sugar.
3. Add cream with the berries.
4. Top it with some dark chocolate shaved chips it you want.
5. Serve it and enjoy.

Chocolaty Coconut Bars

Serves – 15

Cooks In- 20 minutes

Preparation time - 10 min

Difficulty- Easy

Ingredients

- Chocolate Chips – 4 Tablespoon
- Butterscotch Chips – 8 tablespoon
- Peanuts – 8 tablespoon, unsalted
- Coconut Flakes – 7 tablespoon, Sweet and Divided
- Condensed Milk – 14 tablespoon
- Almonds – 4 tablespoon

Method

1. Preheat oven at 375 degree F.
2. Take a baking pan, grease.
3. On to the baking pan, spread more than ½ coconut flakes om the bottom.
4. Sprinkle over the coconut flakes, chocolate chips, butterscotch chips and peanuts.
5. Then add milk over the layer.
6. Finally add rest of coconut flakes and almond.
7. Bake it for 20 minutes.
8. Cool it cut into your desired shape.
9. Serve and enjoy!

Chocolate & Black Bean Brownies

```
Nutrition Facts
Serving Size 101 g
Amount Per Serving
Calories 367              Calories from Fat 150
                                  % Daily Value*
Total Fat 16.7g                          26%
  Saturated Fat 8.9g                     45%
Cholesterol 98mg                         33%
Sodium 141mg                              6%
Potassium 899mg                          26%
Total Carbohydrates 46.0g                15%
  Dietary Fiber 8.5g                     34%
  Sugars 16.4g
Protein 13.2g
Vitamin A 8%           •      Vitamin C 0%
Calcium 11%            •          Iron 20%
Nutrition Grade C
* Based on a 2000 calorie diet
```

Serves – 16
Cooks In- 25 minutes
Preparation time - 20 min
Difficulty- Easy

Ingredients

- Chocolate Chips– 3 oz. Chopped
- Sugar – 7oz.
- Vanilla Extract -1 Tablespoon
- Cocoa Powder – 3.5 oz.
- Olive Oil
- Large Eggs – 6
- Butter – 7 oz., Chopped
- Black Beans – 1 ½ pound ,Rinsed and drained
- Baking powder – 2 Teaspoon
- Salt – ¼ Teaspoon

Method

1. Preheat oven to 375 degree F.
2. In a food processor, add beans, pinch of salt, vanilla, ½ chocolate chips, and 3 pieces of eggs and blend until smooth.
3. Then add butter, cocoa, baking powder, sugar, rest of eggs to the food processor and whisk it until smooth.
4. Prepare a 9 inch baking pan, grease it with oil.
5. Transfer the batter, sprinkle remaining chocolate chips.
6. Bake it for 20-25 minutes in the oven or until tip of knife inserted in the center comes out clean.
7. Cool it cut it into bars.
8. Serve and enjoy!

Peanut Butter Cookie

Nutrition Facts	
Serving Size 129 g	
Amount Per Serving	
Calories 582	Calories from Fat 294
	% Daily Value*
Total Fat 32.7g	50%
Saturated Fat 14.8g	74%
Cholesterol 86mg	29%
Sodium 640mg	27%
Potassium 268mg	8%
Total Carbohydrates 62.5g	21%
Dietary Fiber 2.5g	10%
Sugars 31.1g	
Protein 11.8g	
Vitamin A 12% •	Vitamin C 0%
Calcium 4% •	Iron 25%
Nutrition Grade D-	
* Based on a 2000 calorie diet	

Serves – 5

Cooks In- 15 minutes

Preparation time - 20 min

Difficulty- Easy

Ingredients

- Brown Sugar – 1 cup
- Vanilla Extract -1 Tablespoon
- Peanut Butter – 8 Tablespoon
- Large Eggs – 1
- Unsalted Butter – 8 Tablespoon., Chopped
- GF Flour – 1 ½ cup
- Baking soda – 1 Teaspoon
- Salt – ¼ Teaspoon

Methods

1. Preheat oven for 375 degree F.
2. Take a bowl whisk sugar and butter until soft and fluffy.
3. Add vanilla and eggs, whisk it, then stir in the peanut butter. Toss it properly.
4. Take another bowl; add salt, baking soda, and flour. Mix them.
5. Then add the peanut butter mixture with flour mixture, blend it until evenly mixed.
6. Scoop handful of batter and place on to a cookies sheet.
7. Bake it for 10-12 minutes until it is light brown.
8. Cool it and serve.

Chocolate Pudding with Creamy Orange Zest

Nutrition Facts

Serving Size 112 g	

Amount Per Serving	
Calories 295	Calories from Fat 149

	% Daily Value*
Total Fat 16.5g	25%
Saturated Fat 10.4g	52%
Cholesterol 51mg	17%
Sodium 230mg	10%
Potassium 105mg	3%
Total Carbohydrates 33.9g	11%
Sugars 31.4g	
Protein 2.4g	

Vitamin A 11%	•	Vitamin C 1%	
Calcium 10%	•	Iron 2%	

Nutrition Grade F
* Based on a 2000 calorie diet

Serves – 4
Cooks In- 10 minutes
Preparation time - 15 min
Difficulty- Easy

Ingredients

- Brown Sugar – ¾ cup.
- Chocolate Chips– 1 cup, Chopped
- Heavy Cream – ¾ cup
- Vanilla Extract -1 Tablespoon
- Milk – ¾ cup
- Unsalted Butter – 2 Tablespoon, Chopped
- Orange Zest – ¼ Teaspoon
- Cornstarch – 1 ½ teaspoon
- Salt – ¼ Teaspoon

Method

1. Take a small bowl; add ¼ cup cream, 2 tablespoon sugar and Orange zest . Whisk it using an electric mixer until soft peaks form. Store it in refrigerator.
2. Now take a medium saucepan, mix cornstarch and sugar, stir in cream, salt and milk. Whisk it until it is evenly mixed.
3. Cook the mixture over medium heat, keep stirring until it thickens. Bring it to boil.
4. Remove the pan from heat.
5. Now add vanilla, butter, and chocolate on to the pan, stir it properly.
6. Finally using an electric mixture whisk the mixture until it is fluffy and smooth.
7. Your pudding is ready; divide it into small serving dish.
8. Top it with the refrigerated cream.
9. Serve it and enjoy.

Fruit Cobbler

Serves – 2-4
Cooks In- 40 minutes
Preparation time - 20 min
Difficulty- Easy

Ingredients

- Brown Sugar – ¾ cup.
- White Rice Flour – ¾ cup
- Baking Powder – 1 Teaspoon
- Strawberries -2 Cups , Sliced
- Milk – ¾ cup
- Unsalted Butter – 2 Tablespoon, Chopped
- Peaches – 2 Cups, Sliced
- Salt – ¼ Teaspoon

Method

1. Preheat oven to 375 degree F.
2. Take a large bowl, mix together milk, sugar, salt, baking powder and rice flour.
3. Prepare a 9 inch baking pan, grease it with butter.
4. Add the rice batter into the baking pan.
5. Sprinkle fruits over the batter mixture.
6. Top it with a tablespoon of sugar.

7. Bake it for 35 -40 minutes until it is golden brown.
8. Serve it and enjoy!

Nutrition Facts

Serving Size 268 g

Amount Per Serving	
Calories 343	Calories from Fat 68
	% Daily Value*
Total Fat 7.6g	12%
Saturated Fat 4.3g	22%
Cholesterol 19mg	6%
Sodium 219mg	9%
Potassium 485mg	14%
Total Carbohydrates 66.9g	22%
Dietary Fiber 3.5g	14%
Sugars 39.1g	
Protein 4.6g	
Vitamin A 9% •	Vitamin C 80%
Calcium 15% •	Iron 5%

Nutrition Grade B+
* Based on a 2000 calorie diet

Conclusion

I hope you will use these recipes to create an excellent Cooking Experience for you, your family and loved ones!

I think we should all embrace eating Gluten-Free, healthy and proper food which will help you stay fit and to lose weight (by controlling our insulin and making us less hungry through the day) but also give us oodles of energy to keep going the whole day!

I hope this book was able to help you to satisfy your craving for tasty and delicious food as well as it is GLUTEN-FREE

Part 2

Introduction

The gluten free diet is not a fad diet, it is not a weight loss diet, it is not a "health diet" and it is not a detox diet, no matter what Oprah says. You don't choose to be a celiac or to be gluten intolerant. People who have celiac disease or are gluten intolerant cannot eat gluten without experiencing serious health problems. For other people, gluten is pretty much a neutral substance.

Chapter 1: What is gluten?

1. Gluten, from Latin meaning "glue", is a protein composite found in foods processed from wheat and other related grain species such as barley and rye. Gluten is a composite of a gliadin and a glutenin proteins which gives elasticity to dough, helping it rise and keep its shape and gives it a chewy texture. It is said that gluten was discovered around 7th century by Buddhist monks who were vegetarians and were trying to find a substitute for meat. They discovered that when they submersed dough in water, the starch washed off and all that was left was a meat-like, textured, gummy mass - gluten.

2. Gluten, which literally means glue in Latin, is a protein found in wheat, barley, malt and rye. It is most problematic for individuals with Celiac disease and gluten sensitivity. Since Celiac disease only affects 1% of the population, the likelihood of it is rare, and a lifelong diet free of gluten is necessary. Some of the symptoms of gluten sensitivity, which affects many more people, include; irritable bowel syndrome (IBS), neuropathy (nerve pains and numbness), autoimmune disease, and inflammation. Naturally gluten-free foods are mostly whole foods like fruits, vegetables, nuts, seeds, beans, herbs and wild rice.

3. Gluten is a type of complex protein. Unlike other common proteins, gluten mostly occurs in certain carbohydrates. Wheat, rye etc are rich in gluten.

114

Gluten is an essential component of any bread. It is the reason why bread rises and gains a chewy texture. Gluten makes the bread stretchy.

You hear about the gluten free diet all over - why?

More and more people every day are finding out they have this problem, because at least 90% of processed food - the stuff we all eat every day - contains gluten.

Natural food doesn't have gluten in everything, the way processed food does. Gluten is added in the course of processing for lots of different reasons, including flavoring. What this means is, even if you avoid bread, pastry, pizza, pasta and other obvious sources of gluten (a protein found in wheat, rye, barley and some other closely related grains), you are probably still getting lots of gluten in your food without realizing it.

So it's almost always the case that people who are following a gluten free diet have to go gluten free - although you might be told to "try going gluten free" by your doctor as a diagnostic method, or you might recognize your symptoms match the ones that go with gluten intolerance and decide to try it for yourself.

Living gluten free: it's not easy

So, anyway, assuming you're just starting the gluten free diet - and please read the first paragraph here before you start - it's not that easy.

Like I said before, almost all processed food has gluten in it, to thicken it, to give it a creamy texture, to flavor it, dida dida dida...

There are some very expensive gluten free substitutes for many of the foods you probably take for granted - but even if you can afford them, you might not be pleased with what you get. Many are so vile, I took one mouthful and threw the rest away. Not something I want to repeat too often at the sort of prices we are talking about here.

You know, I used to buy the cheapest pasta - well pasta is pasta, right? 35p a kilo packet, and that did quite a few meals. Now, after trying all the alternatives, I've settled on a nice gluten free pasta brand (Orgran), but that is £1.65 - five timesthe price, for a quarter the quantity. They don't do kilo packs, you can only get a 250g pack. It's priced so high, I often don't put any meat with it any more, just eat it with pesto or a tomato sauce.

I know I'm rambling. Sorry about that. In my next article I will write about cleaning out your kitchen so you have a safe cooking environment for your new diet.

Is the gluten free diet right for you?

If you think you might be gluten intolerant, probably the first step would be the quiz, "Are You Gluten Intolerant?" It's just 5 multiple choice questions and covers things like your symptoms and family history. At the end, you get aresult which is calculated from your answers to all the questions, and you can go from there. If it comes up with a "likely" or "probable" result, you should decide what you want to do next. In the UK, there are good reasons for trying to get a diagnosis of celiac disease - because many special foods can be obtained on prescription.

In other countries, it may be better to just go gluten free on an experimental basis, and see if your symptoms recede. If so, eat something with gluten in it as a test. If your symptoms come back, you've nailed it. The reason I suggest this method, is that it will usually cost you money to get a diagnosis, and there's no clear benefit, since the treatment is just to go gluten free. Why pay money to find out if you shouldn't eat something, when you can just try it and find out for free? In addition, you have to eat a "normal" gluten rich diet for some time before the tests if they are to work.

There's also a "silent" form of celiac disease which is recognized because it doesn't show up in tests, which makes the whole exercise pretty futile in my opinion.

It's not uncommon to hear about people who had celiac disease for 15 years before they were diagnosed correctly. It's a serious matter, because in celiac disease, gluten causes repeated damage to the intestine, which can lead to bowel cancer.

Why is going gluten-free such a hot topic right now?

Because, although Celiac disease only affects 1% of the population, many more individuals are gluten sensitive, which can only be learned by eliminating gluten over a period of 6-months. In fact, 6-10% of the US population has this type of food sensitivity.

Is it healthier to live gluten-free?

There are a variety of products available for anyone who would like to live gluten-free, but like the Standard American Diet, many of the packaged products contain a high amount of sugar, starch and salt. It's very important to be a label detective and review ingredients and note how much sodium and sugars are contained in each serving. Of course the easiest way to have a healthy diet is to concentrate on whole foods including fruit, vegetables, beans, nuts and seeds which are gluten-free naturally. Gluten-free flour is a great product to use when baking, but lacks nutrients typically present in 100% whole wheat flour, so there is no nutrition gained.

Is gluten clearly labeled?

Unfortunately there are not laws that require packaged food to be labeled for gluten content. Some obvious ways to check is to look for any food product containing wheat, barley, rye, brewer's yeast, and beer as well as malt flavoring, malt vinegar and malt. Also, there are cross contamination points with many oats so if you are going gluten-free, only select oats that state they are made in a plant free of gluten. Some of the organic companies will disclose on their packaging that the product was made in a plant that contains wheat, so this is another label to be aware of.

How do I know if I have Celiac Disease?

Celiac Disease can be found by a simple blood test which is almost 100% accurate. Keep in mind that in order for this blood test to accurately identify antibodies you will need to continue eating gluten.

Closing thoughts

Having a diet sans gluten is not for everyone and as you may have guessed, it's difficult to stick to with all the items that do contain gluten like pizza, pasta, and other bread like products as well as crackers and baked and packaged goods. There are several gluten-free substitutes, but they are not a healthier version of an already unhealthy snack or meal. If you are suffering from any of the symptoms listed in the first paragraph of this article, then by all means you should at least speak with a doctor, nutritionist, or health coach about your digestive concerns. Working with a nutrition or medical professional will help you stay on track. These professionals will offer options for alternative foods, healthy gluten-free meals, and can monitor your progress.

Chapter 2: How to Start Becoming Gluten-Free

How to Start Becoming Gluten-Free And Wheat-Free

It's important that we try to stay as healthy as we can, and although this may conjure up images of eating salads and tasteless food, healthy eating is not like this. Healthy eating is all about eating a wide-range of foods that are high in vitamins, minerals and other essential nutrients. These foods will also need to be low in fats, sugar and salt. While we are told to eat wholegrain this and multigrain that, some of these foods could be doing us more harm than good.

This is why you need to think about making your life gluten and wheat-free. Gluten and wheat can have a bad effect on your body, leading to stomach pains, weight loss, constipation, depression and more. If you think you may have a wheat and gluten intolerance then you need to make your life gluten and wheat-free. If you're intolerant or sensitive to wheat then you'll need to eat gluten-free products as the sensitivities are very similar to each other, so for now we'll just concentrate on making your life gluten-free.

Easier Than You Think

It's easier than you think to make your life gluten-free; there are many supermarkets that sell a good range of these foods and you can also find them in some health food stores too.

I know you may think that you're stuck and possibly envisaging a life that consists of eating cardboard-flavored food, but in reality things are quite different.

The next time you go out shopping or decide to shop online, take a look at the great range of gluten-free products your favorite stores sell, I'm sure you'll be impressed.

Cutting down on and cutting out gluten-filled foods is essential to your health and well-being, if you're sensible about it and accept that things are going to have to change, you'll be fine.

From time to time we all crave foods that we can't have, but there's always a tasty substitute somewhere, which makes life a lot more pleasant and satisfying.

There are many support groups that encourage their members to live a gluten-free life, so it's worth considering joining one or two.

Just because you can't eat gluten, it doesn't mean you can't enjoy food anymore, just be sensible, know what you can and can't eat and you'll reap the rewards.

Becoming healthy and staying healthy is so important, which is why you need to think about making your life gluten-free and wheat-free.

Chapter 3: Easy Gluten Free Living

Many people in the world now struggle with Celiac Disease and wonder what to do. Many people want to understand what has happened with their body but more important to them is what do they do now. There are many thoughts that run through people's head so decide they are not going to care about it and try to go on as was but find that they as they go they have more and more complications. Others think they are restricted to only a few select foods and start a diet that is very limited and actually not that healthy. Such diets are believing that you can only eat rice and meat. You do not get all the nutrition that you would need and you would get really bored really quickly because there are only so many combinations of rice and meat.

Going on a gluten free diet does not have to be that limited or restrictive. It at first seems complicated and can seem overwhelming. There are a few tips that can make dealing with Celiac Disease easier.

First is to take it a day at a time. Do not overwhelm yourself by thinking about everything all at once. If you think 'I will never be able to attend this or that because I cannot eat what they will be serving' or 'I will never be able to eat pizza again.' Things like this put you in a negative mind frame and are not helpful in creating a good plan. If you think positively and do not worry too much about how things will be in the future you will find that the gluten free diet will become second nature.

Second is learning to read labels. No, this is not the part of the label that you would check like a diet that is for trying to lose weight. You are looking at the ingredient list and checking for any ingredients that have gluten in them. A lot of products have many ingredients in them with big names. Two things that make it a lot easier than trying to understand all the fancy names that ingredients can have it to just know what to look for. The only ingredients that contain gluten are wheat, barley, rye, oats and all their flours (which will just be their name followed by flour). Also the other one to watch for is barley malt. This is one of the more common ingredients which makes most cereals off the edible list.

Third is to just try different foods and have fun with it. You will find that you like some and not others but it can be a fun experience especially if you do it with someone else. If you do not like something just make fun of it and try something new. There are so many options that you will be able to find a substitute for anything that you could want.

Gluten free living can be handled and can be fun. Think of it as a new and exciting challenge and not a set back or trial. Be patient with yourself, learn a little bit about what you have and what to do. Then have party with it.

Chapter 4: Gluten Intolerance

Mechanism of action

Gluten's action on the gastrointestinal (GI) system has been shown to be complex involving the activation of both the inflammatory and the immune systems.

When gluten containing foods reach the gut, tissue transglutaminase (tTG), an enzyme produced in the intestinal wall breaks down the gluten into its protein building blocks, gliadin and glutenin. One of the other functions of this enzyme is to keep the microvilli in the gut intact.

As gluten proteins pass through the gut, the immune system lining the gut called gut-associated-lymphoid-tissue (GALT) determine if these proteins are potentially safe or unsafe. If recognized as harmful, as in individuals with gluten intolerance, the immune system of the gut produces antibodies against the gluten proteins producing the symptoms of gluten intolerance.

There are two distinct types of intolerance that are ascribed to gluten, namely 'Gluten Sensitivity' and 'Celiac Disease'.

Gluten sensitivity, also known as non-celiac gluten sensitivity, may be best described as a direct reaction to gluten when the body views the gluten protein as an invader and fights it with inflammation both inside and outside the digestive tract.

In celiac disease, on the other hand, the immune system doesn't mount a direct attack against gluten; instead, gluten ingestion triggers the immune system to attack the intestinal lining.

Effects of gluten sensitivity:

The mal-effects of gluten sensitivity on the body as a whole can be diverse and involve many organs. Multiple mechanisms are proposed by different researchers to explain the reason for such a profound effect on the body, some of which are mentioned below.

1- Leaky gut. In gluten intolerant individuals, gluten can cause the gut cells to release a protein called zonulin. Zonulin in turn can break down the intestine's natural protective barrier called tight junction leading to leaky gut syndrome. When the intestine's tight junction is disrupted, undesired substances such as toxins, microbes, undigested food particles and antibodies can leak through to the rest of the body via the blood stream.

2- Autoimmune disorder. When antibodies leak and gain access to the rest of the body then other organs, such as thyroid or brain, are at risk of being attacked by these antibodies, leading to secondary autoimmune disorders.

3- Nutritional imbalance. Since most nutrients are absorbed through the intestinal wall, any damage done to the surface area of the intestinal wall, as is the case with gluten intolerance, can lead to nutritional deficiencies. Such nutritional deficiencies can lead to a vicious cycle of leading to other disease states.

Clinical Symptoms

The symptoms attributed to gluten intolerance vary greatly and many studies are documenting the direct and indirect association of gluten sensitivity with multiple symptoms, signs and disease states. A large number of individuals with gluten intolerance either do not have any symptoms or do not experience any clear cut symptoms. The symptoms of both celiac disease and non-celiac gluten sensitivity are very similar which makes it impossible to determine which type one might have without the use of laboratory tests. The incidence of celiac disease seems to be significantly higher in the elderly than the general population.

The following are some clinical manifestations that in some patients, directly or indirectly, may be associated with gluten intolerance:

1-Digestive issues: Gas, bloating, diarrhea, constipation, irritable bowel syndrome (IBS), Crohn's disease, and ulcerative colitis.

2-Skin and hair issues: Alopecia, eczema, dermatitis herpatiform, and keratosis pilaris, (also known as 'chicken skin' on the back of arms).

3-Autoimmune disorders: Hashimoto's thyroiditis, arthritis, lupus, psoriasis, scleroderma, multiple sclerosis, diabetes, and Sjögren's syndrome.

4-Neurologic symptoms: Ataxia, clumsiness, dizziness, migraine headaches, 'brain fog', and peripheral neuropathy.

5-Nutritional deficiencies: Fat malabsorption, malnutrition, iron deficiency or anemia and vitamin D deficiency.

6-Hormone imbalances: Hypothyroidism, menorrhagia, polycystic ovarian syndrome (PCOS), unexplained infertility, delayed puberty, and short stature.

7-Musculoskeletal issues: Osteoporosis, swelling or pain in joints, bone pain, and muscle spasm.

8-Psychiatric issues: Anxiety, depression, mood swings, ADD, autism, and seizures.

9-Dental and mouth: Teeth with horizontal grooves, oral ulceration and canker sores, dental enamel defect, and bleeding gums.

10-Other symptoms: Body ache, chronic fatigue, fibromyalgia, low energy, weight loss, and urticaria or anaphylaxis in those who use non-steroidal anti-inflammatory medication (aspirin, ibuprofen, etc.)

11-Abnormal laboratory levels: Elevated liver enzymes, low alkaline phosphatase levels.

Causes and contributing factors

Although the cause is unknown, a seemingly sudden increase in the rate of wheat and gluten intolerance has been occurring in the past several decades, forcing researchers to postulate and look for explanations involved in this rapid rise. Gluten intolerance is becoming a major public health issue and according to a Mayo clinic study for example, undiagnosed celiac disease can quadruple the risk of death. Below are some of the proposed causes and contributing factors that may be involved in increasing gluten and wheat intolerance.

1. Consumption of larger amount of gluten. We consume more wheat and other gluten containing foods than before. It is estimated that each American now consumes about 55 pounds of wheat flour every year.

2. Increased craving for gluten. Gluten in the gut is converted into shorter proteins, "polypeptides," called "gluteomorphins." Gluteomorphin (also known as Gliadorphin) is an opioid peptide classified as "exorphins", which act like endorphins and opioids and can bind to the opioid receptors in the brain. They can thus cause addictive eating behavior, including cravings and bingeing. These exorphines have been implicated as a contributing factor, by some neurologist, to some neurological conditions such as depression, ADHD, dementia, schizophrenia and autism.

3. Hybridization. It is referred to a process of combining different varieties of an organism such as wheat to create a particular strain with desirable characteristics, and breed them to reinforce those characteristics. We're no longer eating the wheat that our parents ate.The modern wheat is shorter, browner and far higher-yielding than wheat crops were 100 years ago. Dwarf wheat and semi-dwarf wheat crops have replaced their taller cousins, and these wheat strains reＱuire less time and less fertilizer to produce a healthy crop of wheat berries. The problem is that this hybrid form of wheat produces more gluten than its

ancestors. It is also estimated that 5 percent of the proteins found in hybridized wheat are new proteins that may lead to increased systemic inflammation, widespread gluten intolerance and higher rates of celiac. To make things worse this type of wheat also contains more starch called amylopectin A which is very fattening and increases one's blood sugar significantly. This raise in blood sugar also worsens and fuels an existing inflammatory process.

4. Deaminatetion. Today's wheat has also been deamidated, by acid or enzymatic treatment of gluten, which allows it to be more water soluble. Deamination may produce significant immune response in some people and result in symptomatic gluten-sensitive enteropathy.

5. Genetically Modified Organisms (GMOs). Wheat has been hybridized and not considered a GMO, which by definition is only created by alaboratory process that inserts genetic material into a plant DNA. Some studies, however, link consumption of genetically modified organisms (GMOs) with gluten-related disorders and suggest GMOs might be an important environmental trigger and may exacerbate gluten-related disorders, including celiac disease. Nine GMO foods are being currently grown which constitute as much as 80 percent of conventional processed food in the U.S. They include, soy, corn, cotton (oil), canola (oil), sugar from sugar beets, zucchini, yellow squash, Hawaiian papaya and alfalfa.

6. Genetic predisposition. There are some genes that are found to contribute to gluten sensitivity, mainly human leukocytic antigen (HLA), or HLA-DQ2/8. The presence of these genes makes one more susceptible to developing gluten intolerance.

7. Non-gluten effects of grains. Some of the ill effects of wheat might be contributed to lectin, a non-gluten substance found in wheat and other grains, beans, seeds, nuts, and potatoes. Wheat germ agglutinin (WGA) a non-gluten glycoprotein or lectin is found in highest concentrations in whole wheat and can increases whole body inflammation. It is suggested that lectin-WGA protects wheat from insects, yeast and bacteria. Foods with high concentrations of lectins, may be harmful if consumed in excess. Adverse effects may include nutritional deficiencies, and immune reactions. Possibly, most effects of lectins are due to gastrointestinal distress through interaction of the lectins with the gut epithelial cells.

Incidents

1.It is estimated that celiac disease affects about 1 in 133 people, or close to 1% of the population. However, as few as 5% affected may know they have the condition.

2.Gluten sensitivity, only recently recognized as a stand-alone condition, seems much more prevalent than celiac disease. Some studies estimates that the condition affects 6% to 7% of the population, while other studies place the number as high as 50% of the population.

Treatment

The only treatment for gluten intolerance is strict avoidance of dietary gluten. This requires awareness of obvious and "hidden" sources of gluten in our food as well as awareness of gluten free options.

Gluten containing grains: Wheat, including spelt, Khorasan wheat, faro, durum, bulgur, semolina; Barley; Rye; and Triticale.

Other gluten containing foods: Gluten is often present in other foods such as beer and soy sauce, and can be used as a stabilizing or binding agents in more unexpected food products and medications.

Avoid unless labeled 'gluten-free'

- Beer
- Breads
- Cakes and pies
- Candies
- Cereals
- Cookies and crackers
- Croutons
- French fries
- Gravies
- Imitation meat or seafood
- Matzo
- Pastas
- Processed luncheon meats
- Salad dressings
- Sauces, including soy sauce

• Seasoned rice mixes
• Seasoned snack foods, such as potato and tortilla chips
• Self-basting poultry
• Soups and soup bases
• Vegetables in sauce
• Food additives, such as malt flavoring, modified food starch and others
• Medications and vitamins that use gluten as a binding agent
• Play dough

Gluten free foods.

Many grains and starches, listed below, can be part of a gluten-free diet. You might want to choose those gluten free foods that are labeled non- GMO.

Amaranth
Arrowroot
Buckwheat
Corn and cornmeal
Flax
Gluten-free flours
Hominy (corn)
Millet
Quinoa
Rice
Sorghum
Soy
Tapioca
Teff

Other allowed foods

Many foods are naturally gluten-free including:
Beans, seeds, nuts in their natural, unprocessed form
Fresh eggs
Fresh meats, fish and poultry (not breaded, batter-coated or marinated)
Fruits and vegetables
Most dairy products
How about Oats: There is a great deal of conflicting information regarding the inclusion of oats within a gluten-free diet. Oats are freᐧuently contaminated with wheat during growing or processing which partially explains the different gluten intolerance reactions to oat that can happen. Recent studies indicate that there may also be different amounts of gluten present in different cultivars of oat. For the above reasons oats are generally not recommended.

Diagnosis:

If you have symptoms of celiac (any digestive, allergic, autoimmune or inflammatory disease, including diabetes and obesity) or do not feel well and think that you might have gluten intolerance, you might want to follow the following steps.

1. First find a physician familiar with this condition that can help you diagnose and treat this condition. Please note that in a large number of patients, other issues such as leaky gut, autoimmune reaction, inflammation and nutritional deficiencies must be addressed before the desired outcome is achieved.

2. Rule out celiac disease through celiac disease blood tests or through a small intestinal biopsy.

3. Look for a family history of Celiac disease or gluten intolerance. Check your genes to see if you have the genes that predispose you to gluten (HLA DQ2/8).

4. If the above tests are negative, try a gluten challenge, first eliminating gluten from your diet to see if your symptoms clear up, and then "challenge" it by reinstating it into your diet, to see if symptoms return.

Chapter 5: Gluten Intolerance – "How to Be Gluten Free"

What is it to be gluten free and have celiac disease?

Are you allergic to gluten? Gluten is a protein found in wheat, rye, barley, spelt and triticale. They are prolamins (proteins) that cause damage to the digestive system. Tiny hairlike structures called villi are in the lining of the small intestine. It helps to digest the nutrients in your food. For people who have gluten intolerance or celiac disease, gluten attacks the villi and makes it flat. Then you cannot absorb the nutrients in your food. It is actually an autoimmune disorder. You can also become intolerant to dairy, sugar and possibly other food sensitivities. The only way to reverse the process is to stay away from gluten and the villi will grow back so that you can absorb the nutrients in your food again. Many people can have gluten intolerance or celiac disease and not know it. It is always best to get tested to make sure. I suggest you talk with your primary care physician/G.I. physician to get tested for celiac disease or go to see a nature path to test for food allergens.

What foods contain gluten?

All these foods contain gluten:
Mostly your grains like Wheat, Barley, Barley Malt, Rye, Spelt, Semolina, Graham Flour, Wheat Starch, Wheat

Germ, Couscous, Bran, Kamut, Bulgur, Durum, Triticale, Oats (Oats are not guaranteed from cross contamination, make sure it is gluten free oats)and allot of Alcohol has gluten in it.

So what can you eat in place of gluten?

Non Gluten Flours: Almond Meal Flour, Amaranth Flour, Brown Rice Flour, Buckwheat Flour, Garbanzo Bean Flour, Millet Flour, Potato Starch, Quinoa Flour, Sorghum Flour, Soy Flour, Tapioca Flour/Starch, Arrowroot Flour, and Teff Flour.

Gluten Intolerance Symptoms

These are some of the symptoms of gluten intolerance: Abdominal pain and distension, bloating, diarrhea, greasy foul smelling floating stools, vomiting, acid reflux, constipation, gas and flatulence, nausea, weight loss or weight gain, loss of appetite, fatigue and weakness, headaches and migraines, depression, irritability and mood disorders, fuzzy brain or inability to concentrate, dental enamel deficiencies and irregularities, nerve damage(peripheral neuropathy), respiratory problems, lactose intolerance, rosacea, hashimoto's disease, hair loss, bruising easily, muscle cramping and muscle weakness, swelling and inflammation, vitamin and mineral deficiencies, joint and bone pain, infertility, abnormal menstrual cycles, seizures, ataxia(bad balance), canker sores, eczema and psoriasis, Acne, early onset osteoporosis, night blindness, hypoglycemia(low blood sugar), nose bleeds, elevated liver function tests(AST, ALT), lack of motivation, hashimoto's disease, sjogren's syndrome, lupus erythematosus and other autoimmune disorders, irritable bowel syndrome or spastic colon, inflammatory bowel disease, chronic fatigue syndrome or fibromyalgia, lupus (an autoimmune disease),unexplained anemia, psychological issues(hypochondria, depression, anxiety, bipolar, schizophrenia, neurosis and mood disorders), food allergies, parasites or other infection, gallbladder disease, thyroid disease, cystic fibrosis(respiratory disorder), diverticulosis, diabetes, thyroid Disease, dermatitis herpetiformis(skin rash related to celiac disease), peripheral neuropathy(tingling or numbness in arms and legs), and many more conditions.

Symptoms in children:

Inability to concentrate, irritability, ADD/ADHD or autism and down syndrome, failure to thrive (infants and toddlers), nose bleeds, short stature or delayed growth, delayed onset of puberty, weak bones or bone pain, abdominal pain and distension. If these symptoms are not put under control like being on a gluten free diet, they can turn into more serious conditions. Like heart disease, lung disease, addison's disease, the list goes on and on. Gluten Intolerance and Celiac Disease is an autoimmune disorder.

I am gluten intolerant, now what do I do?

1. See a Doctor, Nutritionist or a Nature Path that, understands what is to be on a gluten free diet.

2. Join a support group like Gluten Intolerance Group. Look up your state and city to find your local support group. You are not in this alone.

3. Find a gluten free blog you really like for tips, recipes and resources.

4. Learn to read food labels. Make sure to look for the gluten free label on grocery products. Learn what what is in your food.

5. Learn how to eat healthy and gluten free, is better for you.

6. Join a gluten free cooking class or find an instructor. Many nature stores have cooking classes.

7. Find your local grocery stores that sells gluten free products. For example, Lingonberries Market, Whole Foods, New Season's, Trader Joe's, Fred Meyer Nutrition Center. Winco, Safeway and Wal-Mart Superstores. There are websites that sell these products. For example, Amazon and The Gluten Free Mall.

8. Find your local Restaurants that are gluten free friendly.

9. Get yourself a couple of Gluten Free Books and a magazine.

10. Search for gluten free coupons online and in the newspaper.

11. Here is a fact you should know, People with Celiac Disease can Declare their "Gluten Free Food" as Tax Deduction.

12. Try different recipes and food products and find out what you like the best. Most of all, have fun with it. Be

sure and avoid cross contamination, you don't want to get gluten mixed up with your non gluten food.

Chapter 6: Living Gluten-Free Is Becoming Easier!

For someone suffering with symptoms of gluten intolerance or celiac disease, living glutino-free does not always seem like an easy alternative. The common perception is that gluten is everywhere! What kind of food options is available to someone with such issues: carrot sticks and cabbage leaves? Fortunately, living gluten-free is becoming exponentially easier with each passing year as more manufacturers, restaurants, and food retailers join this health conscious movement.

The wheat-free, glutino-free industry has posted an annual growth rate of over 25% for the past couple of years. More and more brand name items, such as General Mill's Corn Chex, have the gluten-free symbol proudly displayed on the packaging.

Like all facets of any specialized diet, the burden of shopping for tasty, safe food becomes lighter once you have some experience. You still have to regularly check the ingredient lists and you may need to switch away from some old favorites, but the transition to eating foods safe for the celiac sufferer or food sensitive person is easier than you might think!

Stores such as: Trader Joe's, Whole Foods, Sprouts, & Fresh and Easy are an authentic gold mine of gluten-free products. Also, smaller, neighborhood health and vitamin stores will carry alternative ingredients.

Furthermore, nationwide grocery store chains now allocate an aisle or small section to commodities that do not contain wheat or its byproducts. Also, you can find gluten safe products at larger warehouse stores such as Costco, Sam's Club, or Smart & Final (again, make sure you read the labels)!

As you conduct your own wheat-free research, you will find and ever increasing number of informational resources, cookbooks, and websites to help you live gluten-free. Several food conscious membership sites with forums and regular informational sessions are available on the internet.

Undoubtedly, the safest, surest way to eat without glutino is to cook or bake you own meals. This may sound difficult given that gluten remains hidden in many commonplace foods and ingredients. How, for example, can you bake gluten-free? Switching common ingredients with glutino-free alternatives will allow you to create delicious, safe breads and treats.

Replacing wheat, barley, rye, or spelt with quinoa, millet, buckwheat (despite its name, buckwheat lacks glutino); sorghum, brown rice, almond meal, or potato starch will give you numerous gluten-free baking options. Furthermore, these alternative flours will increase your intake of such beneficial nutrients as calcium, protein, and iron!

The battle to thrive free from wheat and glutino is easier than you imagine. With plenty of resources, ingredients, viable substitutes, and helpful food stores, there has never been a better time to go gluten-free!

Chapter 7: Why Do I Need A Gluten Free Diet?

You've just heard the news from your doctor. Or maybe you've come to the conclusion on your own, perhaps after conflicting medical tests and your unending list of symptoms. Still, this is the moment of truth - you're starting a gluten free diet. The kicker is you have no idea what you're doing. Going low-fat? Cut down on pizza and baby back ribs. Going low sodium? Throw out the salt shaker. Going gluten free? Hmm...canyou repeat thequestion? That's how our family was when my husband had to start a gluten free diet.

We vaguely knew what gluten was, we knew how miserable he felt, but we didn't have any idea how they were connected. And once we heard the news, then what? Was this dramatic change really necessary, and would I have to throw out everything in my kitchen to make it happen? It was a challenge at first, but we survived it. Let me walk you through the basics of what gluten is, where it lurks, what your celiac or gluten sensitivity symptoms might look like, and how gluten can really hurt someone who needs to avoid it.

What Is This Gluten Stuff Anyway?

The first few weeks of grocery shopping after my husband's diagnosis were disorienting and exhausting. Gluten - really? If it jumped off the ingredient label and hit me in the nose, would I know it was gluten? Label-reading can be tough because gluten comes from a handful of different grains and is made into a million different ingredients not labeled as "this looks a lot like gluten." It's a protein found in wheat, barley, and rye. Kneading bread dough activates the gluten protein, creating a strong but flexible structure for the bread. Oats do not technically contain gluten, but it is so often grown and processed near wheat fields that the risk of cross-contamination is pretty good. So-called "clean" oats are grown and processed in isolated fields, with dedicated equipment, and with frequent testing to eliminate this contamination risk.

I Had No Idea Gluten Could Be In That

OK, so you ditch the bread, pasta, donuts, and pizza crust, and that big bag of flour on the back shelf. That'll do it, right? Well, it's a good start, but it's not enough. A gluten free diet goes way beyond the obvious sources. You'll need to crack out your reading glasses and get cozy with food labels from now on. Gluten can be found in malt flavoring (oh no - check nearly any mainstream cereal box), "natural flavoring" (one of those nebulous ingredients near the end of many labels), and random occurrences of
wheat flour (like some potato chips or nut mixes). See what I mean? It's a lot like spotting Waldo in one of those books, except that Waldo sometimes moves around and changes his shirt without telling you.

Feeling Sick In A Hundred Different Ways

Did you hear something about "contamination"? Yes, you did. For some people, gluten is essentially a poison. It is to be avoided completely and consistently. Otherwise, they risk uncomfortable symptoms and potential bodily harm. Gluten sensitivity and celiac disease can share very similar symptoms. But according to current research only celiac disease shows evidence of true intestinal damage. These symptoms can include diarrhea, stomach cramps, marked or unintended weight loss, a "foggy brain" feeling, headaches, general fatigue, abdominal pain, bloating, joint pain, another medical condition seeming worse or failing to improve, depression, irritability, muscle cramps, mouth sores and other dental problems. Children may have stunted growth, "failure to thrive", or may appear sickly and have some of the other symptoms described above. Some have found that behavioral problems and autism have been linked to celiac disease and gluten sensitivity. While this is somewhat controversial and is not yet conclusive, more experts continue to look into the connections.

The list of possible symptoms is a long and winding road, and the end result for each person doesn't always spell something obvious like, "Hey, I have a problem with gluten!" Some have very few, if any obvious symptoms, and it's only confirmed when they get a colonoscopy (often because of some other ongoing medical treatment or evaluation). Others have a wide range of symptoms all the time. You may notice that not all of the symptoms are digestive in nature. The key thing to remember is that a person with true untreated celiac disease is also experiencing malabsorption of nutrients from their food. Food comes in, but their body can't get much from it. Over time, these symptoms or changes develop and take their toll.

Celiac symptoms are commonly overlooked, misinterpreted, mistreated, ignored, or minimized for many years before a proper diagnosis is discovered. And who could blame anyone for taking that long to figure it out? With that wide range of symptoms, problems could be easily written off as harmless issues with no connection to a larger picture. It's not reasonable to assume that any random stomach ache or period of fatigue is automatically the result of a lifelong medical problem. That sounds over-dramatic, right? When it starts to affect your life in a way you can't ignore, that's usually when the pieces fall together. Only when my husband started losing a dramatic amount of weight did we really take action to solve the problem. Once we got the diagnosis and looked in the rear-view mirror, we easily saw the symptoms we'd misread.

Inflammation Is A Very Bad Thing

Here's the biggest reason why anyone diagnosed with celiac disease absolutely needs to avoid gluten at all cost - bodily damage from chronic inflammation. Remember all that about malabsorption of nutrients? The reason that happens is because gluten causes an auto-immune response in the intestines, causing a lot of inflammation. Basically, the body attacks itself when gluten is around. This relentless inflammation causes obvious symptoms like pain and discomfort. It also starts to destroy the villi (tiny finger-like projections that line the digestive tract) that do all the nutrient absorption. As time goes on, the inflammation wears these villi down to a nub. Enter diarrhea, malabsorption, weight loss, fatigue, headaches, and general symptoms of poor nutrition.

Fortunately, there's a way to restore the digestive tract to its original purpose and structure. It's called...the gluten free diet. Yep, that's it. At this point, the complete avoidance of gluten is the treatment. Medication can sometimes help the symptoms, or you may need other treatments while healing up initially. But food is literally your medicine once you get a celiac diagnosis. And for those wondering about gluten sensitivity, you may get any of the above-mentioned symptoms but have no (or very little) evidence of damage to your digestive tract. But even so, who wants to be sick like that all the time? Your body can't function well if it's constantly reeling from symptom episodes and suffering from poor nutrition. In general, the treatment for any level of gluten sensitivity is a gluten free diet.

Gluten Free Diet - It's Good To Be Healthy Again

The entire goal of a gluten free diet is to help your body heal and keep it healthy. Yes, starting out can be confusing and frustrating. Yes, you will likely miss foods you used to eat (that's normal and OK). Yes, you may have to explain yourself for a while until people understand what you're talking about. But through all this, you gain a priceless gift - a healthier body for you to use and enjoy.

If you have other underlying medical problems, you may still have to deal with those. But chances are good you'll manage them better without all the symptoms, inflammation, and nutrient malabsorption. It's a new landscape with ups and downs, but you'll find that you can eat many delicious things on a gluten free diet. It's not like you're being told to go live on the moon (though it may feel like it at first). Every wonderful tasty gluten free food can be found right here on earth.

Conclusion

You have probably heard about gluten free diet and you might be thinking that this is another passing diet fad. But in reality, living gluten free is more than just one of those diet trends that quickly emerge.If you are diagnosed with celiac, the first - and most important - step is to rid your kitchen of any and all foods that contain gluten. This means obvious foods like bread, cookies, cake mixes, pasta, cereal and crackers, and not-so-obvious foods like soups, soy sauce, battered foods and even beer. Start Living Gluten Free Today Carefully plan and research on the meals you eat. It is best to carefully assess all the foods you eat to separate the gluten rich from the gluten free foods. You should go with meals which include vegetables, meat and poultry, fish and fruits as well as dairy and eggs in limited quantities. There are also some other source of protein which are gluten free like tofu, beans and legumes and protein powders. Grains can still be taken but look for gluten free grain products and limit intake per day.

www.ingramcontent.com/pod-product-compliance
Lightning Source LLC
Chambersburg PA
CBHW060233030426
42335CB00014B/1440